Table of Contents

Introduction 1
Secret Key 1: Plan Big, Study Small 2
Secret Key 2: Make Your Studying Count 4
Secret Key 3: Practice the Right Way 6
Secret Key 4: Pace Yourself 8
Secret Key 5: Have a Plan for Guessing 10
Test-Taking Strategies 13
Initiation, Monitoring, and Clinical Management 19
Management of Nutritional Support Outcomes 34
Nutrition Assessment 42
Professional Practice 56
Therapeutic Plan of Care 58
NSC Practice Test 84
Answer Key and Explanations 95
How to Overcome Test Anxiety 110
Online Resources 117

AF834549

Mometrix
TEST PREPARATION

Nutrition Support Clinician

Exam Secrets Study Guide

DEAR FUTURE EXAM SUCCESS STORY

First of all, **THANK YOU** for purchasing Mometrix study materials!

Second, congratulations! You are one of the few determined test-takers who are committed to doing whatever it takes to excel on your exam. **You have come to the right place.** We developed these study materials with one goal in mind: to deliver you the information you need in a format that's concise and easy to use.

In addition to optimizing your guide for the content of the test, we've outlined our recommended steps for breaking down the preparation process into small, attainable goals so you can make sure you stay on track.

We've also analyzed the entire test-taking process, identifying the most common pitfalls and showing how you can overcome them and be ready for any curveball the test throws you.

Standardized testing is one of the biggest obstacles on your road to success, which only increases the importance of doing well in the high-pressure, high-stakes environment of test day. Your results on this test could have a significant impact on your future, and this guide provides the information and practical advice to help you achieve your full potential on test day.

Your success is our success

We would love to hear from you! If you would like to share the story of your exam success or if you have any questions or comments in regard to our products, please contact us at **800-673-8175** or **support@mometrix.com**.

Thanks again for your business and we wish you continued success!

Sincerely,
The Mometrix Test Preparation Team

Need more help? Check out our flashcards at:
http://MometrixFlashcards.com/NutritionSupport

Written and edited by the Mometrix Exam Secrets Test Prep Team
Printed in the United States of America

Introduction

Thank you for purchasing this resource! You have made the choice to prepare yourself for a test that could have a huge impact on your future, and this guide is designed to help you be fully ready for test day. Obviously, it's important to have a solid understanding of the test material, but you also need to be prepared for the unique environment and stressors of the test, so that you can perform to the best of your abilities.

For this purpose, the first section that appears in this guide is the **Secret Keys**. We've devoted countless hours to meticulously researching what works and what doesn't, and we've boiled down our findings to the five most impactful steps you can take to improve your performance on the test. We start at the beginning with study planning and move through the preparation process, all the way to the testing strategies that will help you get the most out of what you know when you're finally sitting in front of the test.

We recommend that you start preparing for your test as far in advance as possible. However, if you've bought this guide as a last-minute study resource and only have a few days before your test, we recommend that you skip over the first two Secret Keys since they address a long-term study plan.

If you struggle with **test anxiety**, we strongly encourage you to check out our recommendations for how you can overcome it. Test anxiety is a formidable foe, but it can be beaten, and we want to make sure you have the tools you need to defeat it.

Secret Key 1: Plan Big, Study Small

There's a lot riding on your performance. If you want to ace this test, you're going to need to keep your skills sharp and the material fresh in your mind. You need a plan that lets you review everything you need to know while still fitting in your schedule. We'll break this strategy down into three categories.

Information Organization

Start with the information you already have: the official test outline. From this, you can make a complete list of all the concepts you need to cover before the test. Organize these concepts into groups that can be studied together, and create a list of any related vocabulary you need to learn so you can brush up on any difficult terms. You'll want to keep this vocabulary list handy once you actually start studying since you may need to add to it along the way.

Time Management

Once you have your set of study concepts, decide how to spread them out over the time you have left before the test. Break your study plan into small, clear goals so you have a manageable task for each day and know exactly what you're doing. Then just focus on one small step at a time. When you manage your time this way, you don't need to spend hours at a time studying. Studying a small block of content for a short period each day helps you retain information better and avoid stressing over how much you have left to do. You can relax knowing that you have a plan to cover everything in time. In order for this strategy to be effective though, you have to start studying early and stick to your schedule. Avoid the exhaustion and futility that comes from last-minute cramming!

Study Environment

The environment you study in has a big impact on your learning. Studying in a coffee shop, while probably more enjoyable, is not likely to be as fruitful as studying in a quiet room. It's important to keep distractions to a minimum. You're only planning to study for a short block of time, so make the most of it. Don't pause to check your phone or get up to find a snack. It's also important to **avoid multitasking**. Research has consistently shown that multitasking will make your studying dramatically less effective. Your study area should also be comfortable and well-lit so you don't have the distraction of straining your eyes or sitting on an uncomfortable chair.

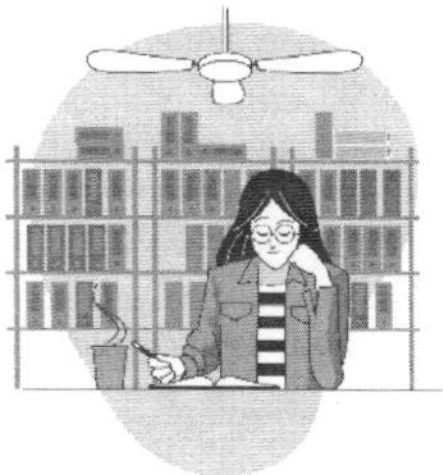

The time of day you study is also important. You want to be rested and alert. Don't wait until just before bedtime. Study when you'll be most likely to comprehend and remember. Even better, if you know what time of day your test will be, set that time aside for study. That way your brain will be used to working on that subject at that specific time and you'll have a better chance of recalling information.

Finally, it can be helpful to team up with others who are studying for the same test. Your actual studying should be done in as isolated an environment as possible, but the work of organizing the information and setting up the study plan can be divided up. In between study sessions, you can discuss with your teammates the concepts that you're all studying and quiz each other on the details. Just be sure that your teammates are as serious about the test as you are. If you find that your study time is being replaced with social time, you might need to find a new team.

Secret Key 2: Make Your Studying Count

You're devoting a lot of time and effort to preparing for this test, so you want to be absolutely certain it will pay off. This means doing more than just reading the content and hoping you can remember it on test day. It's important to make every minute of study count. There are two main areas you can focus on to make your studying count.

Retention

It doesn't matter how much time you study if you can't remember the material. You need to make sure you are retaining the concepts. To check your retention of the information you're learning, try recalling it at later times with minimal prompting. Try carrying around flashcards and glance at one or two from time to time or ask a friend who's also studying for the test to quiz you.

To enhance your retention, look for ways to put the information into practice so that you can apply it rather than simply recalling it. If you're using the information in practical ways, it will be much easier to remember. Similarly, it helps to solidify a concept in your mind if you're not only reading it to yourself but also explaining it to someone else. Ask a friend to let you teach them about a concept you're a little shaky on (or speak aloud to an imaginary audience if necessary). As you try to summarize, define, give examples, and answer your friend's questions, you'll understand the concepts better and they will stay with you longer. Finally, step back for a big picture view and ask yourself how each piece of information fits with the whole subject. When you link the different concepts together and see them working together as a whole, it's easier to remember the individual components.

Finally, practice showing your work on any multi-step problems, even if you're just studying. Writing out each step you take to solve a problem will help solidify the process in your mind, and you'll be more likely to remember it during the test.

Modality

Modality simply refers to the means or method by which you study. Choosing a study modality that fits your own individual learning style is crucial. No two people learn best in exactly the same way, so it's important to know your strengths and use them to your advantage.

For example, if you learn best by visualization, focus on visualizing a concept in your mind and draw an image or a diagram. Try color-coding your notes, illustrating them, or creating symbols that will trigger your mind to recall a learned concept. If you learn best by hearing or discussing information, find a study partner who learns the same way or read aloud to yourself. Think about how to put the information in your own words. Imagine that you are giving a lecture on the topic and record yourself so you can listen to it later.

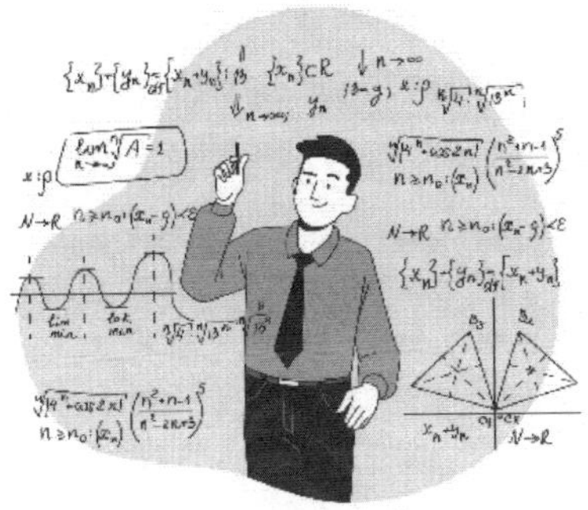

For any learning style, flashcards can be helpful. Organize the information so you can take advantage of spare moments to review. Underline key words or phrases. Use different colors for different categories. Mnemonic devices (such as creating a short list in which every item starts with the same letter) can also help with retention. Find what works best for you and use it to store the information in your mind most effectively and easily.

Secret Key 3: Practice the Right Way

Your success on test day depends not only on how many hours you put into preparing, but also on whether you prepared the right way. It's good to check along the way to see if your studying is paying off. One of the most effective ways to do this is by taking practice tests to evaluate your progress. Practice tests are useful because they show exactly where you need to improve. Every time you take a practice test, pay special attention to these three groups of questions:

- The questions you got wrong
- The questions you had to guess on, even if you guessed right
- The questions you found difficult or slow to work through

This will show you exactly what your weak areas are, and where you need to devote more study time. Ask yourself why each of these questions gave you trouble. Was it because you didn't understand the material? Was it because you didn't remember the vocabulary? Do you need more repetitions on this type of question to build speed and confidence? Dig into those questions and figure out how you can strengthen your weak areas as you go back to review the material.

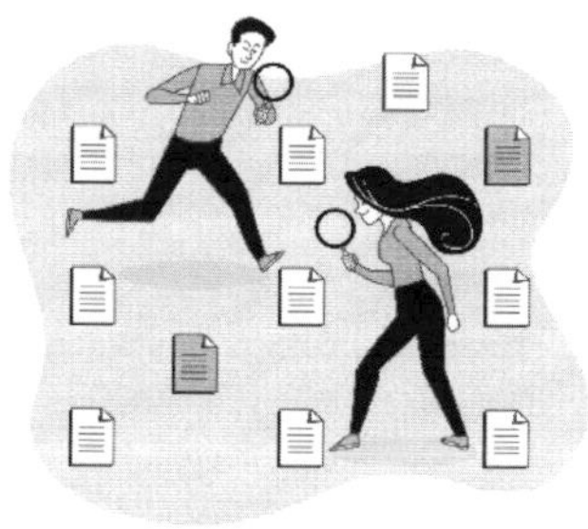

Additionally, many practice tests have a section explaining the answer choices. It can be tempting to read the explanation and think that you now have a good understanding of the concept. However, an explanation likely only covers part of the question's broader context. Even if the explanation makes perfect sense, **go back and investigate** every concept related to the question until you're positive you have a thorough understanding.

As you go along, keep in mind that the practice test is just that: practice. Memorizing these questions and answers will not be very helpful on the actual test because it is unlikely to have any of the same exact questions. If you only know the right answers to the sample questions, you won't be prepared for the real thing. **Study the concepts** until you understand them fully, and then you'll be able to answer any question that shows up on the test.

It's important to wait on the practice tests until you're ready. If you take a test on your first day of study, you may be overwhelmed by the amount of material covered and how much you need to learn. Work up to it gradually.

On test day, you'll need to be prepared for answering questions, managing your time, and using the test-taking strategies you've learned. It's a lot to balance, like a mental marathon that will have a big impact on your future. Like training for a marathon, you'll need to start slowly and work your way up. When test day arrives, you'll be ready.

Start with the strategies you've read in the first two Secret Keys—plan your course and study in the way that works best for you. If you have time, consider using multiple study resources to get different approaches to the same concepts. It can be helpful to see difficult concepts from more than one angle. Then find a good source for practice tests. Many times, the test website will suggest potential study resources or provide sample tests.

Practice Test Strategy

If you're able to find at least three practice tests, we recommend this strategy:

Untimed and Open-Book Practice

Take the first test with no time constraints and with your notes and study guide handy. Take your time and focus on applying the strategies you've learned.

Timed and Open-Book Practice

Take the second practice test open-book as well, but set a timer and practice pacing yourself to finish in time.

Timed and Closed-Book Practice

Take any other practice tests as if it were test day. Set a timer and put away your study materials. Sit at a table or desk in a quiet room, imagine yourself at the testing center, and answer questions as quickly and accurately as possible.

Keep repeating timed and closed-book tests on a regular basis until you run out of practice tests or it's time for the actual test. Your mind will be ready for the schedule and stress of test day, and you'll be able to focus on recalling the material you've learned.

Secret Key 4: Pace Yourself

Once you're fully prepared for the material on the test, your biggest challenge on test day will be managing your time. Just knowing that the clock is ticking can make you panic even if you have plenty of time left. Work on pacing yourself so you can build confidence against the time constraints of the exam. Pacing is a difficult skill to master, especially in a high-pressure environment, so **practice is vital**.

Set time expectations for your pace based on how much time is available. For example, if a section has 60 questions and the time limit is 30 minutes, you know you have to average 30 seconds or less per question in order to answer them all. Although 30 seconds is the hard limit, set 25 seconds per question as your goal, so you reserve extra time to spend on harder questions. When you budget extra time for the harder questions, you no longer have any reason to stress when those questions take longer to answer.

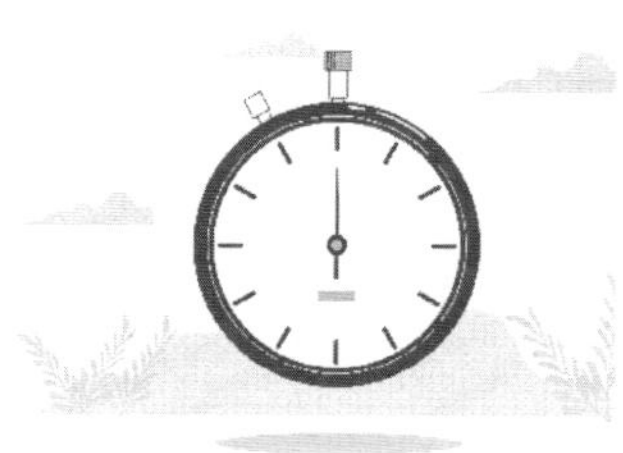

Don't let this time expectation distract you from working through the test at a calm, steady pace, but keep it in mind so you don't spend too much time on any one question. Recognize that taking extra time on one question you don't understand may keep you from answering two that you do understand later in the test. If your time limit for a question is up and you're still not sure of the answer, mark it and move on, and come back to it later if the time and the test format allow. If the testing format doesn't allow you to return to earlier questions, just make an educated guess; then put it out of your mind and move on.

On the easier questions, be careful not to rush. It may seem wise to hurry through them so you have more time for the challenging ones, but it's not worth missing one if you know the concept and just didn't take the time to read the question fully. Work efficiently but make sure you understand the question and have looked at all of the answer choices, since more than one may seem right at first.

Even if you're paying attention to the time, you may find yourself a little behind at some point. You should speed up to get back on track, but do so wisely. Don't panic; just take a few seconds less on each question until you're caught up. Don't guess without thinking, but do look through the answer choices and eliminate any you know are wrong. If you can get down to two choices, it is often worthwhile to guess from those. Once you've chosen an answer, move on and don't dwell on any that you skipped or had to hurry through. If a question was taking too long, chances are it was one of the harder ones, so you weren't as likely to get it right anyway.

On the other hand, if you find yourself getting ahead of schedule, it may be beneficial to slow down a little. The more quickly you work, the more likely you are to make a careless mistake that will affect your score. You've budgeted time for each question, so don't be afraid to spend that time. Practice an efficient but careful pace to get the most out of the time you have.

Secret Key 5: Have a Plan for Guessing

When you're taking the test, you may find yourself stuck on a question. Some of the answer choices seem better than others, but you don't see the one answer choice that is obviously correct. What do you do?

The scenario described above is very common, yet most test takers have not effectively prepared for it. Developing and practicing a plan for guessing may be one of the single most effective uses of your time as you get ready for the exam.

In developing your plan for guessing, there are three questions to address:

- When should you start the guessing process?
- How should you narrow down the choices?
- Which answer should you choose?

When to Start the Guessing Process

Unless your plan for guessing is to select C every time (which, despite its merits, is not what we recommend), you need to leave yourself enough time to apply your answer elimination strategies. Since you have a limited amount of time for each question, that means that if you're going to give yourself the best shot at guessing correctly, you have to decide quickly whether or not you will guess.

Of course, the best-case scenario is that you don't have to guess at all, so first, see if you can answer the question based on your knowledge of the subject and basic reasoning skills. Focus on the key words in the question and try to jog your memory of related topics. Give yourself a chance to bring the knowledge to mind, but once you realize that you don't have (or you can't access) the knowledge you need to answer the question, it's time to start the guessing process.

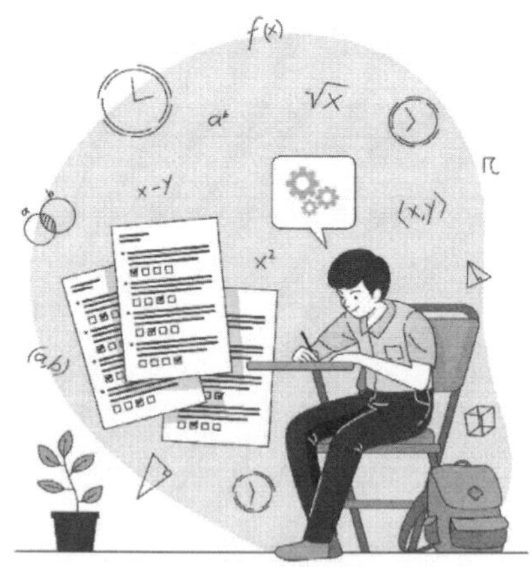

It's almost always better to start the guessing process too early than too late. It only takes a few seconds to remember something and answer the question from knowledge. Carefully eliminating wrong answer choices takes longer. Plus, going through the process of eliminating answer choices can actually help jog your memory.

Summary: Start the guessing process as soon as you decide that you can't answer the question based on your knowledge.

How to Narrow Down the Choices

The next chapter in this book (**Test-Taking Strategies**) includes a wide range of strategies for how to approach questions and how to look for answer choices to eliminate. You will definitely want to read those carefully, practice them, and figure out which ones work best for you. Here though, we're going to address a mindset rather than a particular strategy.

Your odds of guessing an answer correctly depend on how many options you are choosing from.

Number of options left	5	4	3	2	1
Odds of guessing correctly	20%	25%	33%	50%	100%

You can see from this chart just how valuable it is to be able to eliminate incorrect answers and make an educated guess, but there are two things that many test takers do that cause them to miss out on the benefits of guessing:

- Accidentally eliminating the correct answer
- Selecting an answer based on an impression

We'll look at the first one here, and the second one in the next section.

To avoid accidentally eliminating the correct answer, we recommend a thought exercise called **the $5 challenge**. In this challenge, you only eliminate an answer choice from contention if you are willing to bet $5 on it being wrong. Why $5? Five dollars is a small but not insignificant amount of money. It's an amount you could afford to lose but wouldn't want to throw away. And while losing $5 once might not hurt too much, doing it twenty times will set you back $100. In the same way, each small decision you make—eliminating a choice here, guessing on a question there—won't by itself impact your score very much, but when you put them all together, they can make a big difference. By holding each answer choice elimination decision to a higher standard, you can reduce the risk of accidentally eliminating the correct answer.

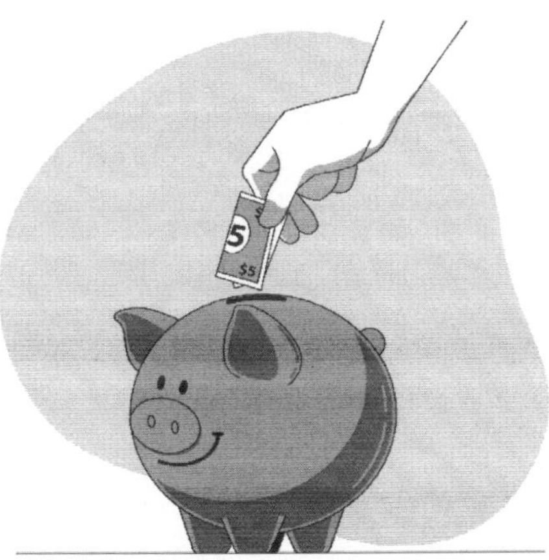

The $5 challenge can also be applied in a positive sense: If you are willing to bet $5 that an answer choice *is* correct, go ahead and mark it as correct.

Summary: Only eliminate an answer choice if you are willing to bet $5 that it is wrong.

Which Answer to Choose

You're taking the test. You've run into a hard question and decided you'll have to guess. You've eliminated all the answer choices you're willing to bet $5 on. Now you have to pick an answer. Why do we even need to talk about this? Why can't you just pick whichever one you feel like when the time comes?

The answer to these questions is that if you don't come into the test with a plan, you'll rely on your impression to select an answer choice, and if you do that, you risk falling into a trap. The test writers know that everyone who takes their test will be guessing on some of the questions, so they intentionally write wrong answer choices to seem plausible. You still have to pick an answer though, and if the wrong answer choices are designed to look right, how can you ever be sure that you're not falling for their trap? The best solution we've found to this dilemma is to take the decision out of your hands entirely. Here is the process we recommend:

Once you've eliminated any choices that you are confident (willing to bet $5) are wrong, select the first remaining choice as your answer.

Whether you choose to select the first remaining choice, the second, or the last, the important thing is that you use some preselected standard. Using this approach guarantees that you will not be enticed into selecting an answer choice that looks right, because you are not basing your decision on how the answer choices look.

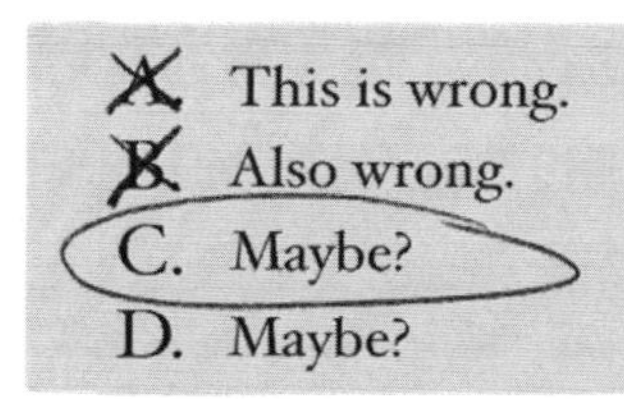

This is not meant to make you question your knowledge. Instead, it is to help you recognize the difference between your knowledge and your impressions. There's a huge difference between thinking an answer is right because of what you know, and thinking an answer is right because it looks or sounds like it should be right.

Summary: To ensure that your selection is appropriately random, make a predetermined selection from among all answer choices you have not eliminated.

Test-Taking Strategies

This section contains a list of test-taking strategies that you may find helpful as you work through the test. By taking what you know and applying logical thought, you can maximize your chances of answering any question correctly!

It is very important to realize that every question is different and every person is different: no single strategy will work on every question, and no single strategy will work for every person. That's why we've included all of them here, so you can try them out and determine which ones work best for different types of questions and which ones work best for you.

Question Strategies

✓ Read Carefully

Read the question and the answer choices carefully. Don't miss the question because you misread the terms. You have plenty of time to read each question thoroughly and make sure you understand what is being asked. Yet a happy medium must be attained, so don't waste too much time. You must read carefully and efficiently.

✓ Contextual Clues

Look for contextual clues. If the question includes a word you are not familiar with, look at the immediate context for some indication of what the word might mean. Contextual clues can often give you all the information you need to decipher the meaning of an unfamiliar word. Even if you can't determine the meaning, you may be able to narrow down the possibilities enough to make a solid guess at the answer to the question.

✓ Prefixes

If you're having trouble with a word in the question or answer choices, try dissecting it. Take advantage of every clue that the word might include. Prefixes can be a huge help. Usually, they allow you to determine a basic meaning. *Pre-* means before, *post-* means after, *pro-* is positive, *de-* is negative. From prefixes, you can get an idea of the general meaning of the word and try to put it into context.

✓ Hedge Words

Watch out for critical hedge words, such as *likely, may, can, often, almost, mostly, usually, generally, rarely,* and *sometimes.* Question writers insert these hedge phrases to cover every possibility. Often an answer choice will be wrong simply because it leaves no room for exception. Be on guard for answer choices that have definitive words such as *exactly* and *always.*

⊘ SWITCHBACK WORDS

Stay alert for *switchbacks*. These are the words and phrases frequently used to alert you to shifts in thought. The most common switchback words are *but*, *although*, and *however*. Others include *nevertheless*, *on the other hand*, *even though*, *while*, *in spite of*, *despite*, and *regardless of*. Switchback words are important to catch because they can change the direction of the question or an answer choice.

⊘ FACE VALUE

When in doubt, use common sense. Accept the situation in the problem at face value. Don't read too much into it. These problems will not require you to make wild assumptions. If you have to go beyond creativity and warp time or space in order to have an answer choice fit the question, then you should move on and consider the other answer choices. These are normal problems rooted in reality. The applicable relationship or explanation may not be readily apparent, but it is there for you to figure out. Use your common sense to interpret anything that isn't clear.

Answer Choice Strategies

⊘ ANSWER SELECTION

The most thorough way to pick an answer choice is to identify and eliminate wrong answers until only one is left, then confirm it is the correct answer. Sometimes an answer choice may immediately seem right, but be careful. The test writers will usually put more than one reasonable answer choice on each question, so take a second to read all of them and make sure that the other choices are not equally obvious. As long as you have time left, it is better to read every answer choice than to pick the first one that looks right without checking the others.

⊘ ANSWER CHOICE FAMILIES

An answer choice family consists of two (in rare cases, three) answer choices that are very similar in construction and cannot all be true at the same time. If you see two answer choices that are direct opposites or parallels, one of them is usually the correct answer. For instance, if one answer choice says that quantity x increases and another either says that quantity x decreases (opposite) or says that quantity y increases (parallel), then those answer choices would fall into the same family. An answer choice that doesn't match the construction of the answer choice family is more likely to be incorrect. Most questions will not have answer choice families, but when they do appear, you should be prepared to recognize them.

⊘ ELIMINATE ANSWERS

Eliminate answer choices as soon as you realize they are wrong, but make sure you consider all possibilities. If you are eliminating answer choices and realize that the last one you are left with is also wrong, don't panic. Start over and consider each choice again. There may be something you missed the first time that you will realize on the second pass.

✓ Avoid Fact Traps

Don't be distracted by an answer choice that is factually true but doesn't answer the question. You are looking for the choice that answers the question. Stay focused on what the question is asking for so you don't accidentally pick an answer that is true but incorrect. Always go back to the question and make sure the answer choice you've selected actually answers the question and is not merely a true statement.

✓ Extreme Statements

In general, you should avoid answers that put forth extreme actions as standard practice or proclaim controversial ideas as established fact. An answer choice that states the "process should be used in certain situations, if..." is much more likely to be correct than one that states the "process should be discontinued completely." The first is a calm rational statement and doesn't even make a definitive, uncompromising stance, using a hedge word *if* to provide wiggle room, whereas the second choice is far more extreme.

✓ Benchmark

As you read through the answer choices and you come across one that seems to answer the question well, mentally select that answer choice. This is not your final answer, but it's the one that will help you evaluate the other answer choices. The one that you selected is your benchmark or standard for judging each of the other answer choices. Every other answer choice must be compared to your benchmark. That choice is correct until proven otherwise by another answer choice beating it. If you find a better answer, then that one becomes your new benchmark. Once you've decided that no other choice answers the question as well as your benchmark, you have your final answer.

✓ Predict the Answer

Before you even start looking at the answer choices, it is often best to try to predict the answer. When you come up with the answer on your own, it is easier to avoid distractions and traps because you will know exactly what to look for. The right answer choice is unlikely to be word-for-word what you came up with, but it should be a close match. Even if you are confident that you have the right answer, you should still take the time to read each option before moving on.

General Strategies

✓ Tough Questions

If you are stumped on a problem or it appears too hard or too difficult, don't waste time. Move on! Remember though, if you can quickly check for obviously incorrect answer choices, your chances of guessing correctly are greatly improved. Before you completely give up, at least try to knock out a couple of possible answers. Eliminate what you can and then guess at the remaining answer choices before moving on.

☑ Check Your Work

Since you will probably not know every term listed and the answer to every question, it is important that you get credit for the ones that you do know. Don't miss any questions through careless mistakes. If at all possible, try to take a second to look back over your answer selection and make sure you've selected the correct answer choice and haven't made a costly careless mistake (such as marking an answer choice that you didn't mean to mark). This quick double check should more than pay for itself in caught mistakes for the time it costs.

☑ Pace Yourself

It's easy to be overwhelmed when you're looking at a page full of questions; your mind is confused and full of random thoughts, and the clock is ticking down faster than you would like. Calm down and maintain the pace that you have set for yourself. Especially as you get down to the last few minutes of the test, don't let the small numbers on the clock make you panic. As long as you are on track by monitoring your pace, you are guaranteed to have time for each question.

☑ Don't Rush

It is very easy to make errors when you are in a hurry. Maintaining a fast pace in answering questions is pointless if it makes you miss questions that you would have gotten right otherwise. Test writers like to include distracting information and wrong answers that seem right. Taking a little extra time to avoid careless mistakes can make all the difference in your test score. Find a pace that allows you to be confident in the answers that you select.

☑ Keep Moving

Panicking will not help you pass the test, so do your best to stay calm and keep moving. Taking deep breaths and going through the answer elimination steps you practiced can help to break through a stress barrier and keep your pace.

Final Notes

The combination of a solid foundation of content knowledge and the confidence that comes from practicing your plan for applying that knowledge is the key to maximizing your performance on test day. As your foundation of content knowledge is built up and strengthened, you'll find that the strategies included in this chapter become more and more effective in helping you quickly sift through the distractions and traps of the test to isolate the correct answer.

Now that you're preparing to move forward into the test content chapters of this book, be sure to keep your goal in mind. As you read, think about how you will be able to apply this information on the test. If you've already seen sample questions for the test and you have an idea of the question format and style, try to come up with questions of your own that you can answer based on what you're reading. This will give you valuable practice applying your knowledge in the same ways you can expect to on test day.

Good luck and good studying!

Initiation, Monitoring, and Clinical Management

Evaluating Home Environment Factors Prior to the Start of Home Nutrition

In order for a patient to be a good candidate for home care nutrition, there are a number of factors that need to be evaluated before therapy can commence. The support system of the patient needs to be evaluated included in the assessment and education. The home needs to have an appropriate electrical source for equipment use. Clean water needs to be readily available for cleaning and for frequent hand washing. The overall condition of the home is also important in relation to cleanliness. Telephone service needs to be readily available for emergency calls and communication with the home care agency and other members of the health care team. A working and clean refrigerator is necessary for the storage of PN solutions that may need to be delivered in 1-2-week allotments. Ideally, a separate refrigerator should be used. Another safety issue that needs to be evaluated is the ability of the patient to safely navigate through their home with equipment.

Impact of Home Parenteral Nutrition

Although home PN can be a lifesaving therapy for many patients, it also requires a major adjustment in lifestyle and routine. Many patients receiving home PN are not debilitated and in fact appear healthy. The addition of home PN can interfere with the patient's ability to work. Often times, the PN schedule created to allow the patient to work interferes with nighttime routines as well. There can be disruptions in sleep patterns due to the infusion process including pump sounds and alarms. It may also cause the need for more frequent visits to the bathroom during the night. Patients who receive home PN also need to adjust to life in a world focused on eating and food. Many patients will try to maintain a normal meal schedule with their family in order to enjoy the social aspect of eating. Others find it difficult to explain why they aren't eating to people outside their family and may need assistance dealing with these types of issues.

Self-Care and Self-Monitoring Components Effective Patient Education

Patient and caregiver education for home PN should begin in the hospital. The initial education stresses the importance of good hand washing and the use of aseptic technique. Home self-monitoring procedures are also taught. This includes 24-hour records for keeping track of all intake and output, urine dipsticks, weight, and temperature. Patients are taught how to interpret these results and when to contact the home care team. Instruction of self-care for the central venous access device is provided as well as dressing change technique. Patient and caregivers should be instructed on safely adding multivitamins or any medications to the home PN bag.

Parenteral Nutrition

Parenteral nutrition can be useful in the following conditions: severe short bowel syndrome, certain types of enterocutaneous fistulas, acute necrotizing pancreatitis, acute flare ups of Crohn's disease, bowel ischemia, obstruction of the lower GI tract, and paralytic ileus. TPN can also be successfully used for malnourished patients who are preparing for surgery. Other indications for PN are for cancer patients unable to tolerate oral or enteral nutrition due to cancer treatments or for critically ill patients unable to tolerate enteral nutrition. The inability to maintain enteral access may also indicate the need for PN. Parenteral nutrition is expensive and can add considerably to the cost of hospital care. Patients should be carefully selected to receive this specialized form of nutrition support.

Total Parenteral Nutrition vs. Peripheral Parenteral Nutrition

TPN and PPN are both ways of delivering nutrition intravenously to a patient who does not have a functioning GI tract. Both forms carry the risk of infection although it is lower for PPN. TPN is delivered through the superior vena cava or other large vein. In this type of vein, blood flows quickly enough to dilute the hyperosmolar solution being infused. Central TPN solutions are typically hyperosmolar because of the glucose, amino acid and electrolyte content. TPN can provide total nutrition to a patient and is indicated for long-term support. PPN is administered through a smaller, peripheral vein therefore the osmolarity needs to be lower to prevent damage to the vein. In order to lower the osmolarity content of the solution, lower amounts of glucose, amino acids and electrolytes will need to be given. Large amounts of fluid are also required to meet calorie requirements. PPN is typically used for a short period of up to 2 weeks

Equipment and Possible Complications for the Patient Receiving Home PN

The patient and caregiver should be educated on how to maintain patency of the catheter. Emergency procedures should be reviewed including what to do if the catheter breaks and how to prevent air emboli form forming. The patient should be instructed on what the symptoms of an air emboli is and what to do if symptoms are present. Training on the use of all home infusion equipment can be done in the hospital initially with follow up at home. The patient should be able to demonstrate proper use of all equipment including set up, administration and disconnection using a regular IV fluid bag. Pump alarms should be reviewed along with troubleshooting for pump issues.

Osmolarity Concerns with Peripheral Parenteral Nutrition

PPN is infused in peripheral veins, which are smaller and less able to handle hyperosmolar solutions. Dextrose needs to be restricted to 5-10% of the final concentration and amino acids need to be restricted to 3% of the final concentration. Final osmolarity should be less than 900 mOsm/liter. Contraindications to PPN include the need for therapy greater than 2 weeks, patients with malnutrition, or patients with liver or kidney disease. It is often difficult to meet the total nutritional requirements of a patient who is critically ill. Patients who require volume restriction, higher amounts of amino acids or certain electrolytes may not be suitable candidates for PPN. Patients must have appropriate veins available for placement of an IV. Phlebitis is a possible complication of PPN related to the osmolarity of the solution.

Cycling Parenteral Nutrition

Cyclic PN refers to an intermittent schedule for administering TPN. Often times, PN will be cycled over 10-16 hours to provide the patient with a period of time off PN. It is also frequently used for patients with cholestatic liver disease related to PN infusion but there is limited research available to document its efficacy. The theory behind this is for the liver to receive a rest from the constant PN infusion. More commonly, cyclic PN is used in the home care setting. This allows the patient more freedom of movement without having to be connected to a pump and IV pole. The patient should have stable blood glucose and electrolyte levels and be able to tolerate a larger rate of infusion. When initiating the cyclic infusion each day, the rate should begin at half the goal infusion rate for the first hour then advanced to the goal infusion rate. This should be followed by a reduction in infusion rate during the last hour of infusion to half the goal rate. This helps to prevent rebound hypoglycemia.

Initiating/Advancing/Discontinuing Parenteral Nutrition

Any irregularities in electrolytes should be addressed before parenteral nutrition (PN) is started. The PN infusion rate can be started at a low volume of approximately 40 cc/ hour in an adult. The patient's vital signs should be closely monitored including blood pressure, pulse, respiratory rate along with blood glucose and other electrolytes. If all are stable, the PN can be advanced to goal within 1-2 days if possible. When the patient is needs to discontinue PN, the rate should be tapered over the last 2 hours to prevent rebound hyperglycemia resulting from the abrupt cessation of the dextrose infusion. An IV dextrose infusion may be substituted to help prevent this. If the patient is transitioning to enteral nutrition and the rate is high enough to support normal blood glucose levels, then the PN does not need to be tapered before discontinuing.

Calculating the Prescription for a Central TPN Solution for a Critically Ill Patient

A full and complete nutrition assessment should be completed ideally by the RD. A working weight needs to be identified for calculating the prescription. Laboratory data should be drawn and examined. Fluid requirements will need to be calculated based on clinical status and hydration needs. Calorie requirements are calculated according to clinical status as well. Next, the macronutrients can be calculated. Dextrose should provide approximately 50-60% of total calories with a maximum glucose infusion rate of 4-6 mg/kg/minute. Amino acids should provide approximately 1.5-2 grams/kg in most cases providing 20-25% of total calories. Lipids should be calculated at 10-30% of total calories with a maximum lipid infusion rate of 0.1 gram/kg/hour. Electrolyte requirements should be determined based on laboratory data and normal requirements. Finally, considerations for multivitamins and trace elements should be reviewed as well as any other possible additives such as medications to the solution.

Propofol in Critically Ill Patients

Diprivan (propofol) is an intravenous sedative commonly used for ICU patients on respirators. The benefit of using this drug is that the dose can be quickly adjusted to achieve the sedation goal and once the drug is stopped, it quickly leaves the system. Propofol is mixed in a 10% lipid emulsion, which can contribute significantly to overall fat intake and must therefore be accounted for when calculating nutritional requirements. This may necessitate the omission of lipids completely from a PN solution if the propofol dose is high enough. Propofol provides 1.1 kcal/ml. Potential side effects of propofol include hypertriglyceridemia related to a decreased clearance of fat. Triglycerides should be checked at least twice per week with goals of less than 400 mg/dl for continuously infused lipids.

Peripheral Access

Peripheral access is determined by the location of the catheter tip outside of a central vein. Peripheral lines are usually placed in veins in the arm or hand or occasionally in the leg or foot. In infants, veins in the scalp are sometimes used for peripheral access. Peripheral lines are for short term use, generally less than 2 weeks. The types of peripheral catheters include standard cannulas, midline catheter and mid-clavicular catheters. A midline catheter is when the catheter tip is advanced 5-7 cm into the upper extremity, however, the tip remains outside of the subclavian vein. This type of catheter can be used up to one month. A mid-clavicular catheter us extended further up into the upper extremity and can be used for up to 3 months.

Selecting the Appropriate Type of Central Venous Access Device

To determine the appropriate CVAD, the patient must first be fully evaluated. The factors to consider in the evaluation process include:

- Clinical status of the patient
- Purpose of the CVAD and length of therapy expected
- Type of IV solution or medication that will be infused
- The training and expertise of the staff who will place the CVAD
- The need for specially trained staff to help care for the CVAD in the hospital or at home
- The patient's ability to participate in care and ability to perform ADL's at home if the CVAD is planned for long term therapy

Features of Central Venous Access Devices

French size refers to the diameter of the outside of the catheter. French size is measured in millimeters. Diameter can refer to both the inside and outside of the catheter. The size of the inside diameter can vary greatly depending upon the material used. Gauge refers to the outside diameter of the needle. The smaller the number of the gauge indicates a larger catheter size. For example, 18-gauge is larger than a 26-gauge needle. A cuff is a term that refers to a device that secures the catheter and helps to prevent any foreign matter from entering the catheter site. Types of cuffs include Dacron, polyethylene or collagen. Lumen refers to separate compartments that have its own connector and port. CVAD can have single, double, triple and quad lumens and these are color coated for safety.

Materials Most Commonly Used in the Production of Central Venous Access Devices

The components used in the production of CVAD are polyvinylchloride (PVC), polyethylene (PE), polyurethane (PU) and silicone. PVC is a rigid material and may increase the risk for forming blood clots and causing phlebitis. PVC may also contain substances that may seep out once inside the body and can cause an inflammatory reaction in the body. PE is commonly used in medically related products. For short term use, PE is durable and is minimally irritating to surrounding tissues. For long term use, however, chronic inflammation may be an issue. PU can increase the risk for clot formation and thus requires the use of anticoagulation therapy if used for more than 24 hours. Silicone elastomer is the most commonly used material. These catheters are soft and supple, and are not likely to cause inflammation.

Contraindications to CVAD Placement

Contraindications to the placement of a CVAD are a fever of unknown origin, neutropenia, or a detrimental change in clinical status. Factors that may impact a safe placement of a CVAD include:

- Patients who have had previously had a CVAD placed need to have their medical history for blood clotting disorders or infection fully evaluated
- Patients who have had shoulder fracture of surgery in the chest or neck region as this may change the anatomy
- Medication use that may affect coagulation ability such as aspirin, heparin, coumadin, or non-steroidal anti- inflammatory medications

Large Veins Used to Obtain Central Venous Access

Large veins such as the superior vena cava (SVC), subclavian, jugular or femoral are all veins that may be used to obtain central venous access. The tip of the catheter should ideally be located in the distal SVC or right atrium. It is important to obtain x-ray confirmation of the placement of line before it is used for any reason. The benefits of central venous access are that by using such a large vein, the blood flow is very rapid and able to handle hyperosmolar solutions and medications. This type of access is for long term therapies. Other benefits include the ability to use this line for drawing blood work, and for transfusions. The risk for central venous access can include infection, pain, pneumothorax, hemothorax, and cardiac arrhythmias.

PICC Line

A PICC line is a peripherally inserted central venous catheter. This means that the line is placed in a peripheral vein but the catheter tip is advanced into the superior vena cava. PICCs are typically inserted in the basilica, cephalic, or brachial vein in the upper part of the arm above the elbow. These are considered non-tunneled catheters, which means the catheter is secured in place by a sterile dressing. The benefit to using a PICC line is that central PN solutions and many medications can be infused safely through the line. A PICC line is less expensive than other types of central access and is easily changed or removed. PICC lines can be used for months and are convenient in both the hospital and home environment. PICC lines can be placed by specially trained staff at the bedside or in radiology. The disadvantage to a PICC line is that the location of the line may interfere with the patient's ability to perform certain activities of daily living such as hygiene.

Implanted Catheters

An implanted catheter (also known as implanted port) refers to a type of device that is implanted under the skin in the chest area. An implanted catheter is placed percutaneously into the jugular or subclavian vein and requires the use of an operating room. A needle is required to gain access to the port, as there is no external tubing for this type of device. The port can be used approximately 2000 times and is used more for intermittent medication administration such as chemotherapy. The advantages to an implanted catheter are that clothing easily conceals it and patients can more easily perform activities of daily living such as hygiene. It is convenient for use in the home setting and carries a lower risk for infection. This type of catheter requires surgical removal.

Tunneled Catheters

A tunneled catheter is a type of central venous access that requires surgical placement under sterile conditions. Two insertion sites are made approximately 6 inches from each other. The first is by near the shoulder and the second is in the mid chest region. The tunneled catheter is placed under the skin then "tunneled" until it reaches the subclavian or jugular vein. By tunneling the catheter, the risk of infection is lower. This type of catheter is used for long term access years in duration if necessary. Advantages of tunneled catheters is that they can be repaired easily if the catheter breaks and the patient is better able to perform activities of daily living such as self hygiene. Disadvantages of tunneled catheters include clotting of the catheter, which will prevent fluid from easily flowing, infection if the site is not kept clean and dry, and thrombosis if a blood clot forms. Types of tunneled catheters include Hickman, Broviac, and Groshong.

Potential Complications Associated with Central Venous Access Devices

The most common complication of CVAD is infection. The cause of infection can be multifactorial and includes contamination of the IV solution being infused into the CVAD, infection resulting from flora normally found on skin, and microbial source at the insertion site. Catheter occlusion is also a commonly seen complication of CVAD. Occlusion is when there is resistance to either the solution being infused or when attempt is made to aspirate blood from the line. The occlusion can be due to thrombosis, intraluminal clotting or mechanical obstruction such as a kinked catheter. A thrombus can be extremely dangerous as it could lead to pulmonary embolism. Air embolism is also a risk and extreme care should be taken not to introduce any air into the catheter. The CVAD can also become dislodged and may require surgical assistance to reposition or replace.

Phlebitis and Extravasation

Phlebitis is defined as the inflammation of a vein. This causes pain, redness, and sensitivity to the area involved. Phlebitis is the most common complication of PPN. To help prevent phlebitis, the peripheral line should be changed to a new location every 2-3 days. Heparin is added to PPN solutions to help reduce the risk. Other ways to reduce the risk is to avoid running any solution with an osmolarity greater than 900 mOsm/liter and concentrated medications such as certain antibiotics. Extravasation occurs when medications being infused intravenously enter into the tissue around the IV site. The risk for extravasation injury is increased with vesicant type drugs that can cause severe injury, burns or blisters to tissue such as chemotherapy drugs.

Causes and Prevention of Intraluminal Clotting of Central Venous Catheters

The most common causes of intraluminal clotting are interactions between certain medications and heparin, PN solutions that have "cracked" or precipitated, and lipid infusion. Occlusions can often be prevented simply by adequate flushing of the catheter using a normal saline flush between all solutions. Careful compounding of the TNA must occur to prevent the occurrence of precipitates. Mechanical blockages can be caused by catheters that are bent, sutures that are too tight, or from a malpositioned clamp. Another type of blockage is called "pinch off" syndrome. This is caused when the catheter is pressed between the shoulder and rib cage because of the way the patient is positioned. Repositioning the patient should open the obstruction.

Monitoring the Critically Ill Patient Starting Parenteral Nutrition

Baseline lab values need to be obtained for the following: electrolytes (sodium, potassium, chloride, CO2), glucose, calcium, phosphorus, magnesium, renal and liver function, albumin, prealbumin or transferrin, complete blood count (CBC) including platelets, and serum triglycerides. Once PN is established, sodium, potassium, chloride, CO2, calcium, phosphorus, magnesium, BUN, creatinine, and glucose should be checked daily for critically ill patients, and the CBC should be checked weekly at the minimum. Liver function tests including ALT, AST, alkaline phosphatase, and total bilirubin should be checked on the first day then weekly. Serum triglycerides should be measured on the first day of infusion after the lipid has infused to check for clearance then should be monitored weekly. The patient's vital signs and clinical status are continuously monitored in an ICU setting. The patient should be weighed daily and close monitoring of all intake including PN and all other fluids being provided such as medications or blood products, and all output including urine, drainage, vomiting, stool, etc. Finally, the catheter site should be checked frequently for any signs of infection.

Transitional Feedings

Transitional feeding occurs when a patient is ready to change from one type of feeding modality to another such as from parenteral to enteral, enteral to oral or parenteral to oral. When a patient is ready to transition from PN to enteral, the tube feeding can begin at ~30 cc/hr. After tolerance has been established, the rate can be advanced by 10-20 cc/hr every 8 hours or as prescribed until a goal rate is reached. There should be a concurrent decrease in the PN infusion rate to keep the caloric intake consistent. Once the patient is tolerating the tube feedings and the volume is providing approximately 75% of the patient's nutrient needs, the PN can be stopped.

Indications for Enteral Nutrition

The term enteral nutrition generally refers to tube feeding. Enteral nutrition is clearly the preferred mode of specialized nutrition support. It is more cost effective than parenteral nutrition. The gold standard for providing nutrition is "if the gut works, use it". Patients must have a GI tract that is working to be eligible. Patients who have malnutrition or are at risk for malnutrition because of poor dietary intake should be considered. Other candidates include patients with an inability to swallow related to a disease process such as cancer or neurological disease. Patients who are critically ill and have increased calorie requirements such as in burns or trauma are appropriate. The ethical considerations for enteral nutrition such as risks and benefits, clinical condition, diagnosis, prognosis, quality of life and the input of the patient and family should be carefully considered before a feeding tube is placed and therapy begins.

Optimal Time to Begin Enteral Nutrition

The ASPEN Clinical Guidelines advise that patients who are well nourished and stable but are unable to receive adequate oral nutrition within 2 weeks or patients who have had inadequate nutrition for 1-2 weeks should begin enteral nutrition. For critically ill patients however, initiation between 24-48 hours following surgery or admission to the ICU may be optimal for better outcomes. Studies have shown that early enteral nutrition may reduce infection rates and lower length of both the hospital and the ICU stay. Early enteral feeding also helps to maintain gut integrity and prevent bacterial translocation. Additional studies need to be done.

Closed System for Enteral Nutrition

A closed system for enteral nutrition involves the use of prepared formulas in ready to hang containers. These containers can hold 500 ml, 1000 ml, 1500 ml or 2000 ml per container. Once the tubing is inserted and connected to the pump, the container can safely hang from 1-2 days. The advantages to this type of system are that it is more cost effective, reduces errors and has lower rates of contamination. The prefilled containers can be stored for long periods of time. It requires less labor to set up the system and provides for more efficient use of caregiver time. One disadvantage is that more waste could occur if the patient does not tolerate the formula and a whole day's supply must be discarded. Other disadvantages are the inability to modify the enteral formula is needed and the possibility of limited product selection depending upon the vendor used for enteral products. Extreme care must be taken that the enteral tubing is connected to the right port as IV administration of an enteral product can cause death.

Open System for Enteral Nutrition

An open system is a system for enteral nutrition that involves a bag or bottle that must be filled before it can be connected to the system. The product used can be ready to feed formulas in cans of boxes or formulas prepared from powder. The advantage to this type of system is that there can be less waste because only what is needed can be prepared and it can also allow for a more tailored nutrition plan for the patient (i.e. diluted tube feeding or modular product use). This type of system also accommodates the use of products that require reconstituting with water. The disadvantage to this system is that there are more chances for contamination because of the number of steps involved, it is less cost effective and requires more labor to set up. The prepared feeding has a shorter hang time because of the risk for contamination.

Contraindications to Enteral Nutrition Therapy

Although enteral nutrition is the preferred mode of nutrition therapy, contraindications do exist. Patients with GI fistulas need to be carefully evaluated for enteral nutrition. Fistulas considered high output and located in the mid jejunum may not be able to be successfully enterally fed. Patients who have had a small bowel resection with less than 100 cm of small bowel left or patients with severe malabsorption should not be enterally fed. Other conditions where enteral nutrition is contraindicated include severe bleeding in the upper GI tract or complete obstruction of the GI tract. Each case should be fully evaluated for the appropriateness of enteral nutrition.

Bolus and Gravity Drip Feedings

Bolus feedings are 240-480 ml of formula are given via feeding tube and large syringe into the stomach over a period of 10-15 minutes. Gravity drip or intermittent feeding is similar to bolus feeding except the volume is placed in a bag or container and infused over a period of 30-60 minutes. Bolus feedings can be given 3-4 times per day while gravity drip feedings are usually given 4-6 times per day. Feedings can be started using 100-150 ml of formula and advanced to the goal volume as tolerated by the patient. Patients who have a normally functioning GI tract can tolerate up to 500 ml per feeding.

The advantages to bolus or gravity drip feedings is that the feeding schedule is flexible and can be tailored to the patient's own routine at home. These types of feeding methods are easier to administer and are lower in cost than feedings delivered via pump. The disadvantages can include tolerance issues because of how quickly a bolus feeding is given or tolerance issues with the amount of volume given. Another disadvantage is that insurance may not cover the extra supplies needed such as bags or tubing. Patients who are at risk for aspiration should not receive either type of feeding method. Patients with feeding tubes placed in the small bowel generally do not tolerate either type of feeding very well.

Continuous Tube Feeding

Continuous tube feedings are tube feedings that are delivered via pump at a designated hourly rate. When continuous feedings are initiated, a low rate of 20-30 ml/hour of full strength formula is used to start. The rate is advanced gradually every 4-8 hours up to goal rate depending upon tolerance and clinical status of the patient. One advantage of continuous feeding is that they are better tolerated than bolus feedings in acutely ill patients. Continuous feedings can be cycled overnight to promote oral intake during the day for patients who are transitioning to an oral diet. Patients who have feedings tubes placed in the small bowel should receive continuous feedings for optimal tolerance. One disadvantage to continuous pump assisted feedings us that mobility may be limited due to the confines of the pump although battery packs are available to increase flexibility. Another disadvantage is more equipment is needed to utilize this method including a pump, tubing, IV pole and a power source. More extensive training is required for using this method of enteral nutrition at home.

Transitioning from Enteral Nutrition to an Oral Diet

Once an enterally fed patient is stable, alert and able to chew and swallow, transition to an oral diet can begin. A Speech Language Pathologist is a valuable resource to use during this transition to diagnose any issues with dysphagia. After the appropriate diet and liquid consistency has been approved and ordered, an oral diet can begin. Tube feedings can initially be held 1-2 hours before meals in order for the patient to feel hungry. Tube feedings can also be cycled at night to help improve the desire to eat and oral intake. As oral intake reaches at least half of the patient's nutritional requirements, tube feedings can begin to be weaned. The amount of formula volume given can be reduced until the patient is consistently able to meet their nutritional needs by oral nutrition solely.

Nasoenteric Tubes

Nasoenteric tubes include nasogastric, nasoduodenal and nasojejunal tubes and are used for short term enteral nutrition of approximately 4 weeks. These tubes can be placed either nasally or orally although nasal placement is more comfortable for the patient after placement. Nasogastric tubes are placed in the stomach and nasoduodenal tubes are placed in the duodenum distal to the pylorus. Nasojejunal tubes need to be placed below the ligament of Treitz. Tubes can be placed at the bedside by staff with appropriate training and expertise, or with the assistance of endoscopy or fluoroscopy. Once placed, the tube should not be used until an x-ray confirms correct placement. Other methods of confirming placement such as pH testing of stomach juices or listening for air pushed through the tube are not recommended. Placement is more successful for nasogastric and nasoduodenal tube tubes than for nasojejunal tubes. Contraindications to nasoenteric tubes would include any mechanical obstruction in the head, neck or throat that would cause harm to the patient during insertion attempts.

Selecting the Proper Type of Tube and Access for Enteral Nutrition Therapy

The type of tube required for enteral nutrition therapy that is needed for 4 weeks or less will generally be a nasoenteric tube. These types of tubes include nasogastric, nasoduodenal or nasojejunal. If longer term access is needed for greater than 4 weeks, a more permanent type of tube should be selected. These tubes will be placed using fluoroscopy, endoscopy, laparoscopy or as an open laparotomy. The type of anesthesia required (i.e. general, local or conscious sedation) should also be carefully considered when selecting how a tube will be placed. The condition of the abdominal wall is an important factor as well as whether the patient has other ostomies, catheters or infusion devices present.

Tube Material

Most nasally placed tubes are made from polyurethane while most percutaneously placed tubes are made of silicone. Silicone is generally a more soft, comfortable tube and is often less stiff than polyurethane tubes. Silicone tubes are less likely to hold their shape when checking for residuals. Polyurethane tubes are usually thinner in diameter and are less likely to erode. Rubber tubes are usually the red type of tubing found in hospitals and latex tubes are the type of tubes used for foley catheters. These types of tubes are not recommended because they breakdown easily and do not have retaining devices to keep them in proper position. The use of latex tubes is also dangerous in the presence of a latex allergy.

Diameter Sizes and Lengths of Various Feeding Tubes

Feeding tubes are available in a multitude of sizes. The diameter of the tube refers to the diameter of the outside of the tube. It does not refer to the diameter of the interior, which can be a factor in how easily a tube will clog. Polyurethane tubes provide a larger inner diameter than other types of tubes. Generally, nasogastric, nasoduodenal and nasojejunal tubes are 8-12 French whereas a gastrostomy tube is 18-28 French, a jejunostomy tube is 8-14 French and a needle catheter jejunostomy is 5-8 French. Lower numbers indicate a smaller diameter. The length of the tube is dependent on where the tube will be placed. A nasogastric tube will be 36 inches whereas a nasoduodenal tube will be 43 inches and a nasojejunal tube will be 60 inches. A guidewire (also referred to as a stylet) is used to provide firmness to a tube while it is being placed through the nose. The guidewire is not as long as the tube in order to prevent puncturing of any part of the GI tract.

Placing a Jejunostomy Tube

A jejunostomy tube can be placed via the direct percutaneous endoscopic method, which is a variation of the PEG procedure. Here the needle is passed through the incision in the abdominal wall and passed into the jejunum. The tube is then passed through the esophagus into the jejunum using the guidewire then threaded out through the original insertion site and secured. A jejunostomy tube may also be placed percutaneously under fluoroscopy. An open jejunostomy is also an option. The Witzel technique is the most common procedure, which involves passing the jejunal tube through a passage created in the submucosa of the small bowel. A needle catheter jejunostomy is an option although it is less popular because the catheter is only 5-8 French and can clog very easily. Jejunostomy tubes can also be placed laparoscopically. One last option is the conversion of a previously placed gastrostomy tube into a percutaneous endoscopic gastrojejunostomy. This basically extends the existing gastrostomy tube into the jejunum.

Placing a Percutaneous Endoscopic Gastrostomy Tube

A percutaneous endoscopic gastrostomy tube (PEG) is a type of feeding tube that is placed endoscopically. Air is blown into the stomach via the endoscope and the appropriate site for insertion is determined. A small cut is made at the site and a needle is passed through the incision into the stomach. A gastrostomy tube is then inserted through the esophagus using a guidewire into the stomach. The tube is then pushed out of the original incision and secured into place using internal and external fasteners. Contraindications to PEG placement are mechanical obstruction located above the stomach and patients who have had gastric bypass procedure. Patients with gastric varices, certain blood disorders, ascites, certain types of cancers in the stomach or abdominal area are not candidates for a PEG. Morbidly obese individuals are also not candidates, as the abdominal wall may not be clearly seen to find an appropriate insertion site due to excess adipose tissue.

Using Clinical Markers to Monitor the Effectiveness of Enteral Nutrition Support

Clinical markers used to evaluate the effectiveness of EN need to be interpreted with care as many are affected by clinical status, fluid status, etc. A physical assessment should be completed including assessing hydration status, weight status, and skin integrity. Vital signs, nutrient intake and output measured from all sources needs to be evaluated. Laboratory monitoring including electrolytes, renal and liver function, CBC, calcium, phosphorus, and magnesium and urine tests should all be evaluated. Assessment of protein adequacy including nitrogen balance and changes in visceral protein stores should be included. Changes in the medication profile should be noted for possible drug nutrient interactions. Assessment of GI function should be also evaluated and overall tolerance to the regimen.

Complications That May Occur During Home Enteral Nutrition

Patient education regarding possible complications for home EN include:

- Prevention and monitoring of dehydration
- Proper skin care and how to identify issues such as skin breakdown, drainage, site infection
- Mechanical complications such as a clogged tube or dislodged tube
- Preventive care such as ways to maintain skin integrity, tube patency and how to prevent the tube from migrating or becoming embedded in the stomach wall
- Securing the feeding tube properly to prevent disconnection during sleep

Enteral Tube Clogging

The most common causes of enteral tube clogging are inadequate flushing of the tube following medication administration, high protein formulations and frequent checking of gastric residuals throughout the day. There are steps clinicians can take to help prevent clogs. Medications can be provided in elixir form if possible although this may cause issues with diarrhea if sorbitol is the base. Any medication provided in pill form should be finely crushed and mixed with approximately 30 ml of water. The tube should be flushed with at least 10 ml of water before and after the medication is given.

Ways to Prevent Clogging and Methods to Unclog These Tubes

Unclogging the feeding tube can sometimes be a simple procedure and other times can be more difficult. The first step is to try to flush the tube with a 60 ml syringe of warm water that is gently pushed back and forth to try to loosen the occlusion. Occasionally, a pancreatic enzyme solution may be administered with a physician order to break up the clog. There are also chemical agents available such as the ClogZapper. Brushes are available that may be threaded through the tube to try to physically break up the occlusion.

Monitoring Plan for Enteral Nutrition in the Hospital vs. Long Term Monitoring at Home

The monitoring plan should include daily intake and output records. The actual amount of enteral formula a patient receives compared to goal should be reviewed at least twice per week. The patient should be weighed 3 times per week or daily is edema or fluid retention is present. Stool output should be monitored daily for amount, consistency, and volume. Electrolytes including sodium, potassium and chloride as well as BUN and creatinine should be checked upon initiation then 2-3 times per week if laboratory values are normal. Blood Glucose, calcium, phosphorus and magnesium should be checked on initiation then weekly unless values are abnormal. Blood Glucose or capillary blood glucose can be checked more frequently if needed. Gastric residuals can be monitored and recorded every 4 hours. For long term enteral nutrition, laboratory testing of sodium, potassium, chloride, BUN, creatinine, glucose, calcium, phosphorus and magnesium should be checked weekly for 4-6 weeks then monthly. If these labs continue to be stable, the labs can be checked every 3 months.

Reasons that Drug- Nutrient Interactions May Occur with the Delivery of Enteral Nutrition

Drug- nutrient interactions can be classified as:

- Physical- where precipitation occurs or causes changes in the viscosity of the formula. Curdling or clumping are also examples.
- Pharmaceutical- where the drug is ineffective because it was not given via the appropriate route

- Pharmacokinetic- where the drug is ineffective or causes toxicity because of altered absorption
- Pharmacodynamic- where the drug is ineffective or cause toxicity because of issues at the binding or receptor sites.

Liquid medications can cause multiple physical interactions due to an acidic pH and certain additives such as syrups, alcohol or oils. Many liquid medications will cause the formula to curdle. Intact protein formulas seem to be fairly incompatible with many liquid medications. Fiber may also play a role.

Drug-Nutrient Interaction for Phenytoin

Phenytoin is a drug used for the treatment of seizures and convulsions. The theory for the drug-nutrient interaction is that there is some sort of binding of phenytoin to either the tubing or to an ingredient in the tube feeding formula. Patients will switch from the IV form to the oral form once enteral nutrition is established. To help maintain therapeutic levels, there are a couple of options for addressing the interaction. One option is to hold the feeding for 1 hour before and 2 hours after phenytoin is given to maximize absorption. Another option is to maintain the normal feeding schedule and increase the dose necessary to reach therapeutic levels. Close monitoring of phenytoin levels are required especially if tube feedings are interrupted.

Impact of Administering the Pill Form of Medications and Enteral Nutrition

If a medication is prescribed in the pill form, there are several considerations to think about before trying to administer via an enteral tube. First, investigate whether the pill can be crushed or dissolved. Examples or medications that should not be crushed or dissolved are slow release, delayed release or sustained release forms. These drugs are usually marked with the following letters: CD, CR, ER, LA, SA, SR, TR, XL, and XR. These pills contain more than one dose per pill and by crushing the pill, the entire day's dose may be given at once causing potentially serious side effects. Certain medications if given all at once can even lead to death. If a pill can be crushed, it should be crushed as finely as possible then added to warm water to dissolve thoroughly before giving the medication through the tube. If the pill is in capsule form, a slurry should be made by mixing the powder and dissolving with water. Once any medication is given. The tube should be flushed with 10 ml of water to maintain patency.

Drug-Nutrient Interaction for Fluoroquinolone Antibiotics

The class of antibiotics called fluoroquinolones include ciprofloxacin, levofloxacin, and ofloxacin. The bioavailability of this type of antibiotic decreases by at least 25% when given with a tube feeding formula. Administration via J tube into the jejunum also has a significant influence on fluoroquinolones and may not be as effective in treating infection if administered this way. This type of antibiotic should not be taken with foods or any meds containing calcium, magnesium or iron because these will bind with the drug. If the patient is receiving tube feedings, the formula should be held for 1-2 hours before and 2 hours after the medication is given to maximize absorption.

Impact of Administering Microencapsulated Products and Enteral Nutrition

If the medication form is a microencapsulated pill containing small beads, these beads may be given via the feeding tube if they are small enough to fit through the tube. Otherwise, the beads should be mixed in an acidic type juice such as orange and given via the tube. The use of the acidic liquid helps to prevent the drug from sticking to the sides of the tube while being administered. Warm water should be used to flush the tube thoroughly after this type of medication is given.

Impact of Administering Enteric Coated & Sublingual Medication and Enteral Nutrition

Enteric coated pills should never be crushed or dissolved in order to give through a feeding tube. These products are coated with a special layer designed to either stop the stomach from becoming inflamed or to stop the breakdown of the pill from gastric acid. If the enteric coat is broken, the patient may not receive the correct dose of the drug or the patient may lose the dose because GI side effect such as vomiting related to irritation. Sublingual medications are small doses of a drug designed to rapidly dissolve in the mouth and are not indicated for administration through a feeding tube. The patient should be able to get the full benefit of the drug sublingually even if the patient is NPO.

Impact of the Administration of an IV or Liquid Form of Medication & Enteral Nutrition

IV forms of drugs are usually the most expensive form and should not be used in the GI tract. IV forms are not designed for exposure to gastric juices and enzymes and may alter or affect absorption. IV electrolytes can be given enterally if needed without any affect to the dose and seem to work appropriately. Liquid drugs for oral use are commonly used but often have a significant osmotic load of greater than1000 mOsm/kg. Using such hypertonic medications in the GI tract increases the chance of the patient experiencing significant GI side effects. Diluting these medications with water will lower the osmolarity slightly but may still be problematic. Also, the use of sorbitol, mannitol, or sucrose for flavoring the medications increases the osmotic load. This osmotic load can be significant when many different medications are given in this form. Sorbitol is especially problematic for causing bloating, gas and diarrhea.

Management of Nutritional Support Outcomes

Refeeding Syndrome

Patients who have malnutrition or who have had an extended period of time without a source of nutrition are at risk for developing refeeding syndrome. Patients with anorexia nervosa and significant alcoholism are also at risk. Refeeding syndrome occurs when nutrition support quickly starts in these patients without giving the body a chance to adjust. It can occur with enteral nutrition but is especially dangerous with the initiation of PN. When the body begins to receive caloric and carbohydrate source too rapidly, the body can respond with serious fluctuations in electrolytes particularly potassium, phosphorus and magnesium because these electrolytes are intimately involved in energy production and tissue growth. The body can also respond with hemodynamic and metabolic instability. Carbohydrate metabolism causes electrolytes to move into the intracellular space as the cells try to utilize glucose for energy. In response to the carbohydrate infusion, the body produces insulin, which causes the body to excrete less water and sodium, which in turn can lead to cardiac or pulmonary failure.

Any patient at potential risk for refeeding syndrome should begin a cautious initiation of nutrition support. Baseline electrolytes and glucose should be evaluated and corrected before initiation. Caloric intake providing less than basal energy requirements with reduced carbohydrate and appropriate amounts of electrolytes should be initiated for the first 24 hours. Electrolytes and glucose should be checked 6-12 hours after PN is started then monitored daily at the minimum and more often if electrolytes are fluctuating significantly so this can be addressed. PN should be gradually advanced to goal for calorie and carbohydrate levels over the next 3-5 days. Provision of electrolytes should be adjusted daily. The patient should also be weighed daily to monitor for fluid overload. Vital signs should be checked frequently.

Hypertriglyceridemia for Patients Receiving PN

Hypertriglyceridemia may play a role in altering the body's immune response and can also lead to pancreatitis. Elevated triglycerides may be due in part to excessive dextrose or lipid infusions. Genetics can also play a role. A baseline triglyceride level should be obtained especially for those with a history of elevated triglycerides or other lipids. In a patient receiving TNA, triglyceride concentrations should be less than 400 mg/dl. If triglyceride levels are greater than 400 mg/dl, the lipids should be omitted from the PN solution. If the IV fat emulsion is piggybacked and run as a separate infusion, it should be administered over 10-12 hours and triglyceride levels should be less than 250 mg/dl 4 hours after the infusion has stopped. To help prevent hypertriglyceridemia, lipids should be limited to 30% of total calories or less or a maximum of 1 gram/kg. The lipid infusion rate should be less than 0.11 gm/kg/hour.

Complications Related to Parenteral Multivitamins Resulting from a Shortage of Multivitamins Solution

Vitamins are required by the body for normal metabolic functioning. Omitting multivitamins from a PN solution can quickly lead to vitamin deficiencies. In the past, nutrition support teams have had to deal with multivitamin shortages. Several deaths occurred as a result of thiamin deficiency. If another parenteral multivitamin shortage occurs, the American Society for Parenteral and Enteral Nutrition has advised that oral multivitamins be used in patients who could tolerate an oral dose. Otherwise, the PN dose should be limited to ~3 times per week. Supplementation of water-soluble vitamins should be given as separate supplements to prevent deficiency as water soluble vitamins have limited stores compared to fat soluble vitamins. Vitamin B12 should be given monthly to prevent deficiency.

Complications Related to Parenteral Multivitamins

Possible complications with parenteral multivitamins include the possible drug nutrient interaction between vitamin K and warfarin. The patient's anticoagulation status must be closely monitored with adjustments made in the warfarin dose as needed. Other complications can include the possible need for additional thiamin supplementation for alcoholic patients or the potential for vitamin A toxicity in patients with renal failure. Lastly, adding the multivitamin preparation to the PN solution too far in advance can lead to complications related to vitamin breakdown. Night blindness has been documented as a result of vitamin A deficiency in patients receiving home PN where the vitamins were not added just before PN administration.

Modifying PN Solutions for a Patient with PN Associated Liver Disease

A thorough reassessment of the patient should be done if clinical signs indicated the development of PNALD. Caloric and dextrose concentrations should be reduced to avoid overfeeding. Less than 70-85% of nonprotein calories should be provided by dextrose. Lipids should be reduced to 1 gram/kg or held. In order to prevent the development of essential fatty acid deficiency, a weekly dose of 500 ml of 20% lipids should be provided for adults. Cycling the PN solution may provide some assistance by reducing the load on the liver. This may help prevent any further progression of PNALD. Manganese and copper should be removed from the PN solution and serum levels should be monitored for deficiency. Carnitine supplementation may help with PNALD because of its role in long chain fatty acid oxidation.

Enteral nutrition should be initiated in patients with PNALD as soon as possible. Trophic levels of jejunal feedings may be beneficial in stimulating bile acid flow. Bacterial overgrowth should be treated with antibiotics. Any sign of infection should be investigated and treated. Medication options are available and have limited success. Ursodiol is the most commonly used medication and it works increase bile flow and help to protect liver cells from the cytotoxicity of the other bile salts. Phenobarbital has also been used although research is scarce to support its use. There is a new option, which shows promise for treating PNALD called omegaven. This is a fish oil based intralipid available only in Europe and under certain conditions in the United States since it is still investigational. For long term PN patients, the only curative option may be intestinal or intestinal/liver transplant. This solution will enable patients to be free from PN support, however, it presents a whole other set of challenges surrounding transplantation of the intestines and/or liver.

Modifying PN Solutions for a Patient with PN Associated Liver Disease

A thorough reassessment of the patient should be done if clinical signs indicated the development of PNALD. Caloric and dextrose concentrations should be reduced to avoid overfeeding. Less than 70-85% of nonprotein calories should be provided by dextrose. Lipids should be reduced to 1 gram/kg or held. In order to prevent the development of essential fatty acid deficiency, a weekly dose of 500 ml of 20% lipids should be provided for adults. Cycling the PN solution may provide some assistance by reducing the load on the liver. This may help prevent any further progression of PNALD. Manganese and copper should be removed from the PN solution and serum levels should be monitored for deficiency. Carnitine supplementation may help with PNALD because of its role in long chain fatty acid oxidation.

Types of Hepatobiliary Disorders Related to PN Therapy

Three types of hepatobiliary disorders associated with PN therapy are:

1. Steatosis where fat accumulates in the liver and may be related to overfeeding. This can present without any symptoms but serum alanine aminotransferase (ALT) and aspartate aminotransferase (AST) will be elevated.
2. PN-associated cholestasis (PNAC) is a disorder that mainly occurs in infants and children and involves impairment in biliary function. Laboratory data will show an elevated direct bilirubin as the primary indicator. Alkaline phosphatase and GGT (gamma-glutamyl transpedtidase) are also elevated. Jaundice may develop. PNAC is very serious as it can lead to cirrhosis and irreversible hepatic failure.
3. Gall bladder sludge or stones can develop causing cholecystitis. The secretion of cholecystokinin is reduced because of the lack of enteral nutrition, which can lead to issues with bile flow and gallbladder function.

Parenteral Vitamin D in the Development of Metabolic Bone Disease

Vitamin D also plays a role in the development of metabolic bone disease. It is recommended that maintenance doses of vitamin D be provided at 200 units as ergocalciferol. Excessive doses of vitamin D can be as dangerous as vitamin D deficiency. Excessive doses can increase serum calcium levels, which can lead to accumulation of calcium in soft tissues such as the kidneys or lungs. Vitamin D deficiency can cause rickets and osteomalacia. In a deficiency state, calcium absorption is not optimized which causes parathyroid hormone to increase leading to increased bone resorption and weakened bones. The presence of liver or renal disease can also affect vitamin D metabolism.

Parenteral Calcium in the Development of Metabolic Bone Disease

Calcium plays an important role in building and maintaining bone mass. Patients on PN are at risk for metabolic bone disease because of reduced calcium as well as increased losses in the urine. Compatibility issues with phosphorus limits the amount of calcium that can be added to PN solutions. When attempts are made to increase parenteral calcium intake, there appears to be a concurrent increase in urinary losses. Other factors that increase urinary losses of calcium include low phosphorus supplementation, chronic metabolic acidosis, and cycled PN solutions. High protein intake also increases urinary calcium excretion. The recommended adult requirement for parenteral calcium gluconate is 10-15 mEq/day with a phosphorus intake of 20-40 mmol/day.

Osteoporosis and Osteomalacia

Osteoporosis and osteomalacia are types of metabolic bone disease that can be related to prolonged use of PN. Osteoporosis is a reduction in bone mass while osteomalacia is softening of the bone due to an impairment in mineralization. The consequences of metabolic bone disease can be bone pain, fractures and a reduction in height due to compression or fractures of the vertebrae. A baseline DEXA scan is recommended for all patients receiving long term PN. Follow up scans can be repeated every 1-3 years depending upon the condition of the bones. Factors in PN solutions that may increase the risk for metabolic bone disease include the adequacy of intake of calcium, vitamin D, magnesium and copper, and possible aluminum toxicity.

Reducing the Risk/Treating Metabolic Bone Disease for Patients with Long Term PN

First, the PN solution should be optimized by providing optimal amounts of calcium, phosphorus, copper, magnesium and vitamin D. Protein should be provided in amounts to meet requirements but not excessively. Avoiding or reducing smoking, caffeine, and alcohol will have a positive impact on bones. Moderate exercise and ambulation are appropriate for weight bearing patients, otherwise, regular physical therapy. Medication options include IV biphosphonate therapy such as pamidronate, selective estrogen receptor modulators such as Raloxifene, calcitonin and estrogen therapy though the use of this should be weighed carefully against the risks. Teriparatide is also available for select patients. This is a synthetic form of parathyroid hormone that acts to stimulate bone formation and increasing bone density.

Concerns for Aluminum and PN

Aluminum is a trace element that has been identified as causing possible toxicity due to its inadvertent presence in certain parenteral products. In 2004, the Food and Drug Administration began requiring manufacturers to label the aluminum content of parenteral products. Approximately 40-75% of any aluminum given parenterally is absorbed. The route of excretion is through the kidneys, therefore, if kidney function is impaired, the risk for toxicity is increased. The consequences of aluminum toxicity can affect the brain by causing neurological impairment.

Aluminum toxicity can affect the bones by impairing bone mineralization leading to osteomalacia. Patients at highest risk for toxicity include patients with renal failure, patients receiving hemodialysis, patients receiving long term PN, and preterm infants and children.

Situations Where Trace Elements Should Be Omitted for Patients Receiving PN

Patients who receive long term PN therapy and have PN associated liver disease (PNALD) should have manganese and copper intake reduced. Excretion of these trace elements is through the biliary tract and this may be altered due to PNALD. Chromium and selenium may be omitted in patients with renal failure, as urinary excretion of both these trace elements may be impaired and lead to possible toxicity. Trace element deficiencies do not happen very often but they can occur in certain situations. Patients not receiving any selenium can develop cardiomyopathy. Zinc deficiency can occur in patients with abnormally high losses such as through drainage from a fistula. Preterm infants need additional zinc for growth.

Management of Blood Glucose During Enteral

The control of blood glucose (BG) levels are of utmost importance especially during critical illness. Avoidance of hyperglycemia helps to prevent fluid shifts related to elevated BG levels and assists with maintaining immune function, which in turn may help with reducing infection rates especially for nosocomial infections. Tight glycemic control has been beneficial in improving morbidity and mortality rates in ICU's. Glycemic control of 80—110 mg/dl is recommended for critically ill patients. The best way to achieve this is through the use of intravenous (IV) insulin. ICU's should have protocols in place for implementing IV insulin therapy and for closely monitoring BG levels with adjustments in insulin according to BG levels. All protocols should include a plan for maintaining BG levels if a tube feeding is interrupted. Some facilities keep a low rate dextrose infusion running while tube feedings are being administered. If tube feedings are held, the dextrose infusion can be titrated up to prevent hypoglycemia.

Etiologies for Nausea and Vomiting in the Enterally Fed Patient

Nausea and vomiting are a common complication of enteral nutrition and can be dangerous as it can increase the risk for aspiration pneumonia or sepsis. Often times, delayed gastric emptying is the reason and the causes for this can be varied. Hypotension, stress, and sepsis can affect gastric emptying. The after effects of anesthesia and surgery can also have an impact of GI function. The use of certain narcotic medications such as morphine or fentanyl can slow GI function. Other medications can cause nausea and vomiting and the side effects of all prescribed medications should be noted. High fat formulas can slow gastric emptying especially if combined with any of the previously mentioned reasons. The rate of infusion or total volume of the bolus as well as the temperature can cause nausea and vomiting in an enterally fed patient. Nausea can also result from the aroma of enteral formulas particularly elemental.

Interventions for the Treatment of Nausea and Vomiting in the Enterally Fed Patient

Appropriate interventions for the treatment of nausea and vomiting include the following:

- Change to an isotonic formula or one that is lower in fat
- Weaning of narcotic medications if able
- Allowing the formula to reach room temperature before it is infused
- Reducing the hourly rate or altering the bolus schedule to provide smaller bolus volumes
- If the aroma bothers the patient, the use of a closed system may help or transition from an elemental to polymeric formula if possible
- Add anti-nausea medications as needed or promotility agents such as metoclopramide or erythromycin

Diarrhea

Diarrhea is a difficult condition to accurately define but indicates watery stool excreted at an abnormal frequency. A more useful definition in the clinical setting is greater than 500 ml of liquid stool per 8 hours or greater than 3 stools per day for more than 2 days. Common causes include:

- Infection including C. Difficile
- Formula intolerance including the fat content or osmolarity
- Lack of fiber
- Medications including antibiotics and sorbitol based elixirs
- Conditions such as short bowel syndrome, HIV, inflammatory bowel disease, bile acid malabsorption, celiac sprue
- Fecal impaction

Medications That May Cause Diarrhea

There are many medications that may cause diarrhea. Antibiotics may be one of the most common. Prolonged use of antibiotics changes or eliminates the normal gut flora potentially leading to bacterial overgrowth. Commonly used antibiotics that may cause diarrhea include ampicillin, clindamycin, penicillamine, neomycin and erythromycin. Sorbitol based elixirs can also cause diarrhea as the sorbitol acts as an osmotic diuretic drawing water into the bowel. Common elixirs that contain sorbitol are tylenol, tagamet, lasix, indocin, and reglan. Lactulose causes diarrhea and is often prescribed for this reason in patients with elevated ammonia levels. Magnesium based medications can cause diarrhea. Other medications to consider include digoxin, hydralazine, methotrexate, procainamide, and theophylline. One last consideration would be if a medication is administered via a jejunal tube. These drugs are often hypertonic and may cause a dumping like condition if given jejunally.

Treatment of Diarrhea in an Enterally Fed Patient

First the cause of the diarrhea should be identified. This includes stool samples to rule out any pathogens. If an enteric pathogen such as C. diff is identified, treatment should be started immediately. The medication should be reviewed for potential diarrhea causing medications and provide substitutions if able. Treatment can otherwise include a change to a fiber containing formula or adding a source of soluble fiber. Sometimes a simple change in type of tube feeding provided is helpful with the control of diarrhea. If C. diff has been ruled out, an antidiarrheal agent can be added. The last step is usually a trial of an elemental or peptide based formula. Of this does not work, bowel rest may be indicated with the initiation of PN until the diarrhea resolves.

Constipation

Constipation is infrequent excretion of stool. Constipation is difficult to quantify because normal defecation varies between individuals. Constipation can be clinically defined as a buildup of waste in the colon that can also include the transverse colon or cecum. An x-ray is needed to verify constipation and rule out other conditions such as an obstruction. Dehydration is a common cause of constipation and care should be taken to provide adequate hydration especially to the elderly and those with limited mobility. Inadequate fiber intake can be a cause and once a fiber source is added, adequate fluid needs to be provided to prevent recurrence. A good bowel regimen is essential to hospitalized patients especially those in the ICU. For patients that are able to move around, exercise and walking around also promote normal, regular bowel movements.

Pulmonary Aspiration

Pulmonary aspiration is the inhalation of foreign substances into the lungs. Aspiration can cause many types of lung infections including pneumonia, pneumonitis, bronchitis, empyema, and can lead to the development of adult respiratory distress syndrome (ARDS). Risk factors for developing aspiration pneumonia include improper positioning of the patient during tube feeding delivery such as lying flat. Level of alertness, neurological impairment or neuromuscular diseases can contribute to the risk. Other risk factors include delayed gastric emptying, vomiting, a history of aspiration, and improperly placed feeding tubes. The symptoms of aspiration are difficulty or rapid breathing, fever, wheezing, and abnormal breath sounds. Pulmonary aspiration sometimes exhibits no symptoms and is referred to as silent aspiration.

Detecting Pulmonary Aspiration

Pulmonary aspiration can be difficult to detect and diagnosis often depends on the presence of symptoms after the tube feeding is vomited or regurgitated. X- rays do not typically show aspiration although if the patient has symptoms and there is evidence of a new lung infiltrate, then aspiration can be presumed. Adding blue food coloring to the formula has been a common practice in many institutions, however, this raises the possibility of allergic reactions to the dye, bacterial contamination of the formula, or causing inaccurate guaiac testing. The Food and

Drug Administration issued a health advisory in 2003 because blue food dye #1 was found to have permeated various body parts, organs and fluids potentially causing death to several patients. This method should no longer be used especially in critically ill or acutely ill patients. One last method for monitoring for aspiration is the use of glucose oxidative strips. This method has not been shown to be sensitive enough to detect aspiration of enteral formulas.

Interventions That May Help to Reduce the Risk for Pulmonary Aspiration

Patients who are at high risk for pulmonary aspiration should be identified and closely monitored. Keeping the head of the bed elevated to 45 degrees during tube feeding can reduce reflux of gastric contents. Gastric residuals are also a commonly used tool for monitoring; however, research has not shown a correlation between high gastric residuals to vomiting, gastric emptying, or pneumonia. The gastric residual volume considered to be elevated varies between institutions. The residual volume can also vary greatly depending upon the position of the patient or type of feeding tube. It is best to monitor and record residuals and watch for a pattern in individual patients rather than interrupting nutrition based on one arbitrary volume of gastric residual. Gastric residuals greater than 200 ml should be carefully evaluated looking for the presence of abdominal distention, nausea, and to ensure safety measures are in place.

Tube Feeding Syndrome

Tube feeding syndrome is a term that refers to dehydration. This is often caused by the provision of excess protein intake and insufficient fluid to help the kidneys excrete the excess urea. Laboratory values will likely reflect an elevated sodium and blood urea nitrogen. A rule of thumb for calculating fluid requirements is 1 cc of water for each calorie provided.

Problem

Calculate how much additional free water is needed for the following patient: A 75 kg stable patient receiving 2160 cc per day of a standard, polymeric fiber containing formula. List additional factors that will influence hydration requirements.

Solution

The patient is receiving approximately 2160 kcals per day thus would need approximately 2160 cc of water per day. The tube feeding is providing approximately 84% free water or a total of 1814 cc per day. This patient would require an additional 346 cc of water per day, which could be divided 3 or 4 times throughout the day to flush the tube. Additional factors that may increase fluid needs would be excess sweat, a hot, humid environment and fever. Feeling thirsty and concentrated urine are also signals for additional water.

Nutrition Assessment

NUTRITION FOCUSED PHYSICAL ASSESSMENT

A nutrition focused physical assessment utilizes a variety of data to provide a complete nutritional assessment of a patient. The physical exam is conducted by a trained practitioner and is entered into the medical record. The exam generally starts at the head and works downwards to the feet.

- Overall appearance, height, weight, wasting
- Vital signs
- Skin - color, integrity, wounds, overall condition
- Nails -color, size, shape, clubbing, texture
- Head - shape, presence of temporal wasting, condition of hair, masses
- Eyes - color, condition, sclera, conjunctiva, ability to see at night
- Nose and mouth - shape, condition of skin, teeth and gums,
- Neck - masses, range of motion
- Cardiovascular and pulmonary - presence of edema, wasting, breath sounds, presence of IV catheters
- Abdomen - color, wounds, feeding tubes, bowel sounds
- Kidney - color of urine and laboratory data
- Musculoskeletal -condition of arms and legs, joint pain, muscle loss, swelling, amputations, range of motion
- Neurological - gross and fine motor skills, level of alertness

HEIGHT

Height is needed to determine Ideal Body Weight (IBW) or Desired Body Weight (DBW). Self reported heights are often inaccurate as are visual estimations made by a practitioner. A patient can be measured using the alternate methods:

- Height measuring scale- generally mounted on a wall
- Arm span- the patient stands with back against a wall, heels together and stretches his arms out sideways. The distance between the tips of both middle fingers is measured.
- Summation of body parts- often used with a patient who is immobile. The heels, legs, pelvic area, spine, and head are measured using a soft measuring tape. The measurements are then added together.
- Knee Height- the formula for calculating knee height is below
- Men: Height (in cm) = 64.19- (0.04 x age [in years]) + (2.02 x knee height [in cm]
- Women: Height (in cm) = 84.88 – (0.24 x age [in years]) + (1.83 x knee height [in cm]

Body Mass Index

BMI is a ratio of weight to height and provides an estimation of body fat. The BMI can be overestimated for athletes with a higher amount of fat- free mass or can be underestimated for those who have lost muscle mass such as the elderly. The equations for calculating BMI is as follows:

- Weight (kg) ÷ Height2 (meters squared)
- Weight (pounds) ÷ height2 (inches squared) x 703

BMI is classified according to the following table:

$$
\begin{aligned}
> 40 &= \text{Obesity Grade III} \\
35 - 39.9 &= \text{Obesity Grade II} \\
30 - 34.9 &= \text{Obesity Grade I} \\
25 - 29.9 &= \text{Overweight} \\
18.5 - 25 &= \text{Normal Weight} \\
17 - 18.4 &= \text{Protein Energy} \quad - \text{Malnutrition Grade I} \\
16 - 16.9 &= \text{Protein Energy} \quad - \text{Malnutrition Grade II} \\
< 16 &= \text{Protein Energy} \quad - \text{Malnutrition Grade III}
\end{aligned}
$$

Hamwi Method for Estimating Ideal Body Weight

The Hamwi Method of quickly calculating IBW was published in 1964. It is also known as "rules of 5's and 6's". It uses the following equation:

- Men= 106 pounds for the first 5 feet of height plus 6 pounds for each inch over 5 feet
- Women= 100 pounds for the first 5 feet of height plus 5 feet for each inch over 5 feet.
- A range of 10% is used to accommodate differences in frame size.

Using IBW in hospitalized patients is difficult because is does not take into account weight change or comparison to usual weight. Also, IBW does not take into account if a patient has had an amputation. Often times, there is edema or anasarca present, which adversely affects weight. There are other methods for estimating weight that measure fat free mass such as tricep skinfold measurements (TSF), or bioelectrical impedance analysis (BIA). Lean Body Mass can be measured using mid arm circumference or mid arm muscle circumference.

Calculating IBW for an Amputee

The equation for estimating IBW for an amputee is as follows:

- Estimated IBW= [(100 - % of amputation) / 100] x estimated IBW for pre-amputation height

The following table discusses the percentages for various body parts to adjust the IBW:

Body Part	Percentage
Head and Neck	8
Trunk without limbs	50
Hand	0.7
Forearm without hand	1.6
Forearm with hand	2.3
Upper arm	2.7
Entire arm	5
Foot	1.5
Lower leg without foot	4.4
Lower leg with foot	5.9
Thigh	10.1
Entire leg	16

For example, a patient with a left below the knee amputation whose pre-amputation IBW was 190 pounds would have an adjusted IBW of approximately 179 pounds.

$$\text{Estimated IBW} = (100\% - 5.9\% \div 100\%) \times 190 \text{ pounds} = 178.8 \text{ pounds}$$

Diet History Tools

Three common tools are a 24-hour recall, a food diary or food record and a Food Frequency questionnaire. A 24-hour recall requires the use of an interviewer with experience obtaining the necessary information. Information obtained from the patient includes any food or beverage consumed in the prior 24 hours and the amounts. A food diary is a record of food consumed over a 1-7 day period. The patient is required to estimate or weigh portion sizes for more accuracy. The patient needs to be able to read and write in order for this tool to be effective. A food frequency questionnaire (FFQ) takes the most time to complete. FFQ estimates caloric and nutrient intake. The patient must report how often a food or beverage is eaten over the course of a predetermined period of time (i.e. a week or a month). This tool is often used in large epidemiological studies.

Electrolytes, Water, Vitamins and Minerals

The function of Vitamin D is for the regulation of calcium and phosphorus levels, and for promoting bone health. Vitamin D also helps with immune function. Vitamin D can be consumed in the diet or produced through exposure to sunlight. Serum 25 hydroxyvitamin D is hydroxylated in the liver and is the main form of Vitamin D in circulation. Serum 1,25- dihydroxyvitamin D is the second hydroxylation that occurs in the kidney. This is the physiologically active form of Vitamin D and is also called calcitriol. Serum calcium, serum phosphorus, and parathyroid hormone regulate this form of Vitamin D. Signs of Vitamin D deficiency include rickets in children and osteomalacia in adults. Vitamin D deficiency can be caused by advanced age, inadequate intake, inadequate exposure to sunlight, liver or kidney failure, fat malabsorption, and short bowel syndrome. Certain medications can also cause a deficiency such as anticonvulsants, corticosteroids or cimetidine. Infants who are exclusively breastfed and do not receive supplemental Vitamin D are also at risk for deficiency.

Causes and Signs of Deficiencies

Thiamin- most common cause of deficiency is alcoholism, inadequate intake, refeeding syndrome, conditions with increased needs such as pregnancy or hyperthyroidism, dialysis, diarrhea, fever, gastric bypass, folate deficiency. Clinical symptoms include beri-beri, peripheral neuropathy, poor memory, Wernicke Korsakoff syndrome (encephalopathy, mental confusion, listlessness), tachycardia, heart failure, and anorexia.

Riboflavin- causes of deficiency include alcoholism, inadequate intake, elderly, malabsorption, and conditions with increased needs such as pregnancy, trauma or burns, biliary obstruction, liver disease, diabetes mellitus. Clinical signs include cheilosis, red tongue, and dermatitis.

Niacin- causes of deficiency include alcoholism, malabsorption, and conditions with increased energy needs such as pregnancy, burns, and trauma. Clinical signs include pellagra (dermatitis, dementia, diarrhea, death), glossitis, stomatitis, abdominal discomfort, nausea, vomiting

Pyridoxine (B6)- causes of deficiency include alcoholism, inadequate intake, liver disease, malnutrition, riboflavin deficiency, conditions with increased needs such as pregnancy, dialysis. Clinical signs include dermatitis, glossitis, stomatitis, confusion, and peripheral neuropathy.

Magnesium

Magnesium- magnesium is involved in over 300 biochemical reactions in the body including carbohydrate and fat metabolism, energy transport, protein synthesis and adenosine triphosphate activity, enzyme function, bone and tooth formation, and active transport of calcium and potassium across cell membranes. Magnesium also affects nerve impulse conduction, muscle contraction and normal cardiac function. Magnesium helps maintain normal blood glucose levels. Deficiency of magnesium can be caused by alcoholism, diarrhea, vomiting, malabsorption, advanced age, renal disorders. Loop and thiazide diuretics can also deplete magnesium. Magnesium level should be checked in patients with low serum calcium or potassium. Signs of deficiency include loss of appetite, muscle cramps and weakness, tingling, numbness, abnormal heart rhythms. Signs of magnesium toxicity are similar to those of magnesium deficiency and include nausea, diarrhea, abdominal cramping, decreased appetite, muscle weakness, change in mental status, irregular heartbeat and difficulty breathing. There is a higher risk of toxicity in patients with renal failure due to the inability to excrete magnesium. Laboratory tests include serum magnesium level and urinary excretion.

Iron

The function of iron includes synthesis of hemoglobin and red blood cells, energy metabolism, oxygen transport, and normal brain development. Causes for deficiency include inadequate intake, use of low iron infant formula without additional iron supplementation, excessive milk intake in place of iron rich foods, long term TPN, malabsorption, prolonged blood loss, pregnancy, menstruation, use of epoetin without iron supplements, chronic use of aspirin, non-steroidal drugs or steroid use. Symptoms of iron deficiency include lack of energy, lethargy, irritability, pale skin, pica, spoon shaped nails (koilonychia), microcytic hypochromic anemia, compromised growth and development in children. Signs of toxicity include constipation or diarrhea. IV or IM iron can cause an anaphylactic reaction. Common lab tests include hemoglobin, hematocrit, serum ferritin, serum iron, Total Iron-Binding Capacity (TIBC), transferrin saturation, mean corpuscular volume (MCV).

Selenium

Selenium functions in the production of antioxidant enzymes, which assist in preventing cellular damage from free radicals and helps with immune function. Signs of selenium deficiency include cardiomyopathy, muscle pain and weakness, and reduced immunity. Deficiency can occur in malabsorption, diarrhea, selenium free TPN solutions, rapid growth without adequate intake. Selenium toxicity may present as changes in hair texture, changes in nails, dermatitis, peripheral neuropathy, and irritability. Laboratory tests used to evaluate selenium status are plasma selenium and glutathione peroxidase. Plasma selenium is affected by recent intake but may not reflect actual stores.

Copper

The function of copper is as a component of many enzymes, cellular metabolism, formation of connective tissue, and iron metabolism. Copper deficiency can occur with inadequate intake especially in preterm or low birth weight infants, malabsorption, cystic fibrosis, advanced age, and inadequate intake in TPN or diet. Signs of deficiency are microcytic anemia, low reticulocyte count, skeletal abnormalities, changes in the pigmentation of hair and skin. Signs of toxicity include nausea, vomiting, diarrhea and abdominal pain. Plasma copper or ceruloplasmin levels evaluate copper status though these tests reflect short-term stores.

Zinc

Zinc functions as a component of over 100 enzymes and for DNA synthesis. Zinc is needed for wound healing, immune function, and growth. Zinc is important for taste and smell acuity. Causes of zinc deficiency include alcoholism, malabsorption, increased losses such as burns or open wounds, renal losses such as nephrotic syndrome, inadequate intake in TPN or poor diet. Deficiency signs include loss of appetite, poor wound healing, dermatitis, changes in taste or smell acuity, poor growth, hair loss, decreased levels of alkaline phosphatase, hypogonadism. Signs of zinc toxicity can include low copper stores, decreased immune function, and reduced levels of HDL cholesterol. Laboratory tests used to evaluate zinc status include plasma zinc level, alkaline phosphatase activity and urinary zinc excretion. Low plasma zinc levels can be related to hypoalbuminemia.

Function of Phosphorus in the Body

Phosphorus plays a major role in energy production through adenosine triphosphate (ATP) and creatine phosphate. DNA and RNA contain phosphorus related compounds. Phosphorus plays a role in bone and teeth formation, muscle and nerve contraction, and renal function. It is involved in growth and the repair of cells and tissues through its role in protein synthesis. Phosphorus also acts as a buffer and assists with acid base balance. Hypophosphatemia occurs when serum phosphorus is less than 3.0 mg/dl. Refeeding syndrome, starvation, severe alcohol abuse, poor phosphorus intake either through diet, intravenous fluids or TPN solution can all cause hypophosphatemia. Other causes include diarrhea, malabsorption, vomiting and increased urinary losses. Vitamin D deficiency, burns, anabolism, diabetic ketoacidosis (DKA), respiratory alkalosis, and hyperparathyroidism can be reasons for low serum phosphorus.

Function and Regulation of Potassium in the Body

Potassium is the main cation in the intracellular fluid. Potassium helps to maintain fluid balance in the body, assists with cell growth, helps to control the activity of muscle tissue such as skeletal, heart or smooth muscles found in the intestines. Potassium is absorbed in the small intestine. 80-90% of potassium is excreted in the urine. The kidneys are responsible for maintaining normal serum values. Hypokalemia occurs when serum potassium is less than 3.0 mEq/Liter. Insufficient intake, alcohol abuse, diarrhea, vomiting and fistula losses, and eating disorders such as anorexia nervosa can cause hypokalemia. Hypokalemia can also be caused by inadequate aldosterone production and Cushing's syndrome. Symptoms can include nausea, vomiting, muscle weakness, paralysis, changes in EKG, T wave alterations and arrhythmias. Certain medications may cause potassium depletion including loop or thiazide diuretics such as lasix or chlorathiazide, insulin, cisplatin, and amphotericin B.

Hyperkalemia

Hyperkalemia occurs when serum levels are greater than 5.0 mEq/Liter. This can be caused by chronic renal failure, increased intake of potassium in the setting of poor kidney function, massive tissue necrosis, burns, rhabdomyolysis. Diabetic ketoacidosis can cause hyperkalemia. Potassium sparing diuretics such as spironolactone, and beta-blockers such as propanolol can cause hyperkalemia as well as potassium supplements. Mild hyperkalemia can often have no evident symptoms but the patient may have muscle weakness, irregular heartbeat or irregular pulse. Severe hyperkalemia will likely have changes in EKG. Cardiac arrest is a possible consequence if left untreated. Treatment includes a potassium restriction. Intravenous fluids and insulin are given to move the potassium from the serum back into the cells. Loop or thiazide diuretics may be provided to promote potassium excretion. Other medications such as Kayexalate are given to bind potassium and cause excretion through stool. Dialysis may be an option if other methods are not effective in reducing potassium levels.

Hypernatremia

Hypernatremia occurs when serum levels are greater than145 mEq/Liter. Serum sodium is more reflective of fluid status than of sodium intake. Causes of hypernatremia can include insufficient water intake, increased water loss from the kidney due to loop diuretics such as Lasix, acute tubular necrosis, or Diabetes Insipidus. Hypernatremia can also be due to an osmotic diuresis related to hyperglycemia. Vomiting, diarrhea, excessive sweating, and burns can also cause hypernatremia. Hypernatremia occurs frequently in the elderly population. Signs of hypernatremia initially can be thirst or dry mouth. Symptoms can progress to confusion, listlessness, fatigue, seizures, and eventually death if not treated. These symptoms are caused brain cell shrinkage. Treatment includes correction of free water deficit in the body with caution to not correcting too quickly to prevent cerebral edema and permanent brain damage. Fluids can be given orally if the patient is able to tolerate or can be given intravenously. Serum osmolality should also be monitored while correcting hypernatremia.

Calcium

Calcium is required for normal bone and teeth formation. It also plays a role in muscle contraction, nerve conduction, and blood clotting. It helps to regulate the heart. Bones and teeth contain approximately 99% of the total body calcium. The extracellular fluid, blood and tissue cells contain the remaining 1%. Calcium from the bones is in a constant state of flux between the bone, blood and extracellular fluid. Calcium is absorbed in the small intestine with the majority absorbed in the ileum. Vitamin D (1,25 dihydroxy vitamin D form) controls the absorption of calcium at the brush border. Passive absorption of calcium, which is not dependent on vitamin D for absorption, occurs in the small intestine and accounts for most the calcium that is absorbed from the diet. The amount of dietary calcium available is inversely related to how efficiently the mineral is absorbed.

Calcium in the bones is in a constant state of flux with the blood and the extracellular fluid. Parathyroid hormone (PTH) regulates serum calcium levels. When serum levels fall, PTH stimulates the release of calcium from the bone into the blood stream. PTH also influences resorption of calcium in the kidneys. Other hormones such as calcitonin and estrogen also play a role in calcium regulation. Total serum calcium is made up of approximately 48% of ionized or free calcium. Protein bound calcium and complexes between calcium and other anions such as citrate make up the rest. Because serum calcium is protein bound, serum levels are decreased with hypoalbuminemia. Ionized calcium is the best indication of the amount of calcium physiologically available in the body.

Hypocalcemia

Hypocalcemia is defined as a serum level less than 9.0 mEq/dl or an ionized level less than 4.5 mg/dl though standards may vary slightly between labs. Symptoms of hypocalcemia increase in intensity as serum level decreases. Symptoms can include muscle cramps, numbness or tingling in the hands, fingers, feet or lips and changes in mental status. Severe hypocalcemia can cause tetany, EKG changes, seizures and convulsions. Hypocalcemia can be caused by low albumin level since calcium is protein bound, hypoparathyroidism, vitamin D deficiency, osteomalacia, liver failure and kidney failure. Other lab values that can affect serum calcium levels are hyperphosphatemia and low serum magnesium. Medications such as corticosteroids, anticonvulsants such as phenobarbital and phenytoin, loop diuretics such as lasix, and calcitonin can all decrease calcium levels.

Hypercalcemia

Hypercalcemia is defined as serum calcium level greater than10.5 mg/dl or ionized calcium greater than 5.6 mg/dl though standards can vary between labs. Symptoms of hypercalcemia start to occur when serum levels are greater than11.5 mg/dl and can include nausea, vomiting, changes in mental status, changes in EKG. Hypercalcemia can cause loss of appetite, excessive thirst, excessive urination leading to dehydration, and muscle weakness. Soft tissue deposits can occur in chronic cases of hypercalcemia and hyperphosphatemia where the calcium phosphorus product is greater than 70 mg/dl. In severe hypercalcemia (serum level greater than 18 mg/dl), renal failure, coma or death can occur. Certain types of cancer such as breast, lung and kidney can cause hypercalcemia as well as multiple myeloma or metastatic bone cancer. Hyperparathyroidism and hyperthyroidism both can cause elevated serum calcium. Medications such as thiazide diuretics, lithium, and excessive vitamin D intake can also cause hypercalcemia. Excessive calcium intake and lack of mobilization can contribute.

Essential Fatty Acid Deficiency

Essential Fatty Acids (linoleic and linolenic) must be obtained from food, as the human body cannot synthesize them. EFA are needed for maintaining skin, cell membranes, synthesizing prostaglandins and leukotrienes. Symptoms of EFAD are a scaly dermatitis/generalized rash, hair loss, thrombocytopenia, and poor growth. Long term EFAD can impair brain and retinal development. Deficiency is rare but can occur if less than 2-4% of calories are provided are from linoleic acid. EFAD can occur in the following cases:

1. Prolonged period of time receiving lipid free TPN
2. Infant fed a formula that does not provide enough EFA such as a medium chain triglyceride (MCT) based formula
3. Severe fat malabsorption following intestinal resection

Laboratory tests used to diagnose EFAD are serum eicosatrienoic acid (triene) level which is a non essential fatty acid that will be elevated in EFAD and serum arachidonic acid (tetraene) level that will be decreased. Triene to tetraene ratio will be greater than 0.2- 0.4 to indicate deficiency. Deficiency can develop within 1-3 weeks.

Function of Water in the Body

The function of water in the body is for temperature regulation, the excretion of waste products from the body, the delivery of nutrients and to help with multiple pathways for energy production. Water is required for digestion and absorption. Water maintains both intracellular fluid, which is the fluid within cells, and extracellular fluid. Extracellular fluid contributes approximately 33% of the total body water and consists of the water found in plasma, lymphatic fluid, spinal fluid and bodily secretions. Total Body Water content averages ~60% but can range from 50-70% depending upon lean body mass. The DRI for water is 30 ml/kcal or a minimum of 1500 ml per day. Hospitalized patients usually require 30-35 ml/kg per day but can vary according to fluid status.

Dehydration

In dehydration or under- hydration, the patient may experience a reduction in the following vital signs: cardiac output, blood pressure, central venous pressure and pulmonary artery wedge pressure. The patient may experience an elevation in body temperature and heart rate. Urine will be concentrated. Weight loss may occur. The eyes and mouth will be dry and the eyes will appear sunken. The skin will be cool to the touch. The patient may show signs of confusion. Possible causes of dehydration include fluid intake that is less than the body's requirements either through not enough IV fluid, inadequate fluid provided through tube feeding or the patient is not drinking enough. The body may lose too much fluid through excessive vomiting or urine or stool output, excessive losses through a nasogastric tube or ostomy. Elevated losses can also occur with fistulas, dialysis, open wounds, and burns. Insensible losses can occur through fever or excessive sweating. Chronic diseases such as kidney disease or cystic fibrosis may increase risk. Various medications can also cause dehydration.

Fluid Overload

A patient with fluid overload will likely have weight gain greater than 1 kg/day and edema throughout the body including the legs and facial/orbital area. The patient may have trouble breathing due to fluid accumulation around the lungs. Blood pressure, heart rate and cardiac output will be increased as well as central venous pressure and pulmonary artery pressure. Causes of fluid overload or over-hydration include fluid received during surgery or resuscitation, poor renal function, impaired liver function causing ascites, congestive heart failure or pulmonary edema. Patients will often be fluid overloaded following cardiac surgery that involved cardiopulmonary bypass. Fluid overload can also occur with the syndrome of inappropriate anti-diuretic hormone secretion (SIADH). Third space fluid refers to fluid that is accumulating in the extracellular and extravascular spaces causing generalized edema. Fluid overload is treated with diuretics with a sodium and/or fluid restriction. Paracentesis may be indicated for patients with ascites.

Function and Regulation of Sodium in the Body

Sodium is the main cation in the extracellular fluid. Sodium helps to control the volume of extracellular fluid and plasma. Sodium also plays a role in the conduction of nerve impulses and muscle contraction. Sodium is absorbed in the intestines then is filtered and returned back to circulation by the kidneys. Aldosterone, which is secreted by the adrenal cortex, helps to regulate sodium balance. Hyponatremia can be caused by the syndrome of inappropriate antidiuretic hormone secretion (SIADH), through increased losses through the skin or lungs, fluid overload from congestive heart failure or pulmonary edema, or glucocorticoid deficiency. Hyponatremia occurs when serum level is less than125 mEq/Liter. Signs can include nausea, vomiting, headache, muscle pain, disorientation, disagreeable and feeling sluggish or tired. In severe cases, coma or death can occur if untreated.

Albumin, Transferrin, Prealbumin, and Retinol Binding Protein as Visceral Protein Indicators

Albumin, transferrin, retinal binding protein, and pre-albumin are all negative acute phase proteins. This means that the liver produces less of these proteins in response to inflammatory stress. Albumin is found in the serum and has a long half-life of approximately 20 days. It is the most plentiful plasma protein. Because of its long half-life, albumin does not respond rapidly in patients receiving nutrition support. Albumin level is affected by fluid status and liver function. Transferrin is a plasma protein with a half-life of approximately 8 days. It is more responsive to nutrition support; however, synthesis of transferrin increases when iron stores are low and may not always be reflective of protein stores. Prealbumin is also called transthyretin and is responsive to short term changes in nutritional status because its half-life is only 2 days. Zinc deficiency will affect synthesis of prealbumin. Retinol binding protein is a plasma protein with a half-life of 12 hours. Studies have shown that it correlates well with protein status.

Nitrogen Balance

Nitrogen balance is used to assess the adequacy of protein status. A 24-hour urine collection is necessary.

To calculate:

$$\text{Nitrogen balance} = \text{Nitrogen intake} - \text{Nitrogen output}$$

To calculate nitrogen intake, divide grams of protein intake by 6.25 to convert protein to nitrogen.

To calculate nitrogen output=

$$\text{Urinary urea nitrogen (mg/100 ml)} \times \text{urinary volume (L/day)} / 100 + 20\% \text{ of urinary urea losses} + 2 \text{ grams}$$

Healthy adults have a zero nitrogen balance. A negative nitrogen balance can be seen in starvation, protein energy malnutrition, critical illness, and hypermetabolism. A positive nitrogen balance is seen in growth, pregnancy and anabolism. Factors that can affect how accurate the study are: impairment in kidney function, inaccurate collections, and additional nitrogen loss in stool or in ostomy output.

Function of Protein in the Body and Essential Amino Acids

Protein is required for growth in children and adolescents. It is required for almost all parts of the body including muscles, organs and skin. Protein is a component of enzymes, hormones, and antibodies. It can be used as a source of energy if there is not enough carbohydrate or fat present in the diet; however, it is used at the expense of growth, tissue repair and maintenance. Protein is made up of amino acids and the body needs 20 amino acids for protein synthesis. 13 of these amino acids are called non-essential because the body can synthesize them. There are 9 amino acids that are essential because the body can't synthesize them. They must be obtained through the diet. Essential amino acids are isoleucine, histidine, leucine, lysine, methionine, phenylalanine, threonine, tryptophan, and valine.

Metabolic Acidosis and Metabolic Alkalosis

Metabolic acidosis occurs when there is excess acid or lack of base. This can occur when the kidney does not excrete enough hydrogen ions. Metabolic acidosis can be further categorized by whether there is an anion gap. Metabolic acidosis can occur with lactic acidosis, diabetic ketoacidosis (DKA), renal failure, liver failure, an overdose of salicylate, or ingestion of ethylene glycol. Diarrhea or other losses from the GI tract can also cause metabolic acidosis. Laboratory data will show a low pH and serum $HCO3$ level and a normal $PaCO2$.

Metabolic alkalosis occurs when there is a deficit of acid or an excess of base (bicarbonate). Metabolic alkalosis can occur with suctioning of the GI tract, vomiting, abuse of laxatives, use of diuretics or volume depletion. It can also occur when too much base is provided such as in the form of citrate or acetate, use of Ringer's Lactate solution, or excessive antacids. Laboratory data will show an elevated pH and serum $HCO3$ with a normal $PaCO2$.

Maintaining Acid-Base Balance in the Body

Acid-base balance is maintained in 3 ways.

1. Through a buffer system which generates a quick response to changes in pH level. The buffer system uses proteins, phosphates, bicarbonate, and carbonic acid to normalize pH levels.
2. Through the kidneys that control the reabsorption of bicarbonate and the excretion of hydrogen ions to help keep the plasma bicarbonate at the correct concentration.
3. Through the lungs that regulate respiratory function to adjust the amount of carbon dioxide exhaled.

The goal of acid base balance is to keep the blood pH level at 7.35- 7.45. Alterations can occur due to different disease states, medications, and fluid imbalance and can be threatening if not treated. The other lab data used to evaluate acid base balance is $PaCO2$ (partial pressure of carbon dioxide) and serum bicarbonate ($HCO3$).

Respiratory Acidosis and Respiratory Alkalosis

Respiratory acidosis occurs when breathing is decelerated and carbon dioxide retention occurs. Respiratory acidosis can be caused by brain injury, primary hypoventilation syndrome, pneumonia, sleep apnea and obesity. It can also occur with alterations is neuromuscular function such as with multiple sclerosis, myasthenia gravis, brain stem injury, muscular dystrophy, or amyotrophic lateral sclerosis (Lou Gehrig's disease). Cardiac arrest and sever pulmonary edema can also be causes. Laboratory data will show a low pH level and an elevated PaCO2 level while serum HCO3 level could be normal or slightly elevated.

Respiratory alkalosis occurs when breathing is quickened and too much carbon dioxide is exhaled. Respiratory alkalosis can occur in patients who are over-ventilated while on a respirator. Respiratory alkalosis can be caused by pneumonia, early acute respiratory distress syndrome (ARDS). It can be due to too little oxygen being circulated related to high altitude level or from anemia. It can be triggered by an effect on the central nervous system such as a stroke or a brain tumor or from anxiety leading to hyperventilation. Laboratory data will show an elevated pH level, a low PaCO2 level while serum HCO3 will be normal.

Stool Studies

Fecal Leukocyte

Fecal leukocyte test shows whether there are white blood cells (WBC) present in the stool. Presence of WBC can indicate bacterial infection or an inflammation such as a type of colitis. WBC will not be present in stool with a viral or non-infectious illness.

Ova and Parasites (O & P)

Ova and parasite test checks for the presence of parasites or eggs. This is generally used to determine the cause of infection if there is a history of international travel or exposure to a potentially contagious environment such as a daycare center.

Occult Blood

Occult blood is a test that looks for the presence of blood in a stool that is not obvious to the eye. A positive test can indicate an infectious process or cancer.

Clostridium Difficile Toxin (C. Diff)

Clostridioides difficile checks for the presence of toxin in the stool sample. C. Difficile infection is commonly seen in patients receiving antibiotics greater than 2 weeks. Symptoms of c. diff infection include diarrhea, abdominal pain, fever, and leukocytosis. If symptoms persist after a negative culture, additional stool samples should be obtained and tested.

Fecal Fat

Fecal fat test is a test that checks for the presence of malabsorption. The patient needs to consume 80-100 grams of fat per day for three days. Stool is collected for 72 hours to check for absorption. Less than 7 grams of fat present in stools in a 24-hour period is considered normal.

Normal Growth

Infants generally gain approximately 30 grams per day in the first 4 months. The rate of weight gain decreases to approximately 10-20 grams per day through the first year. Infants normally double their birth weight by 4 months, then triple their birth weight by 12 months of age. Typical weight gain is approximately 2-3 kg per year up until age 9-10. Weight gain will continue to increase as puberty approaches. Birth length will increase by 50% in the first year but will not double until approximately 4 years. Height will increase by 6-8 cm per year up until puberty. A major growth spurt will occur around the time of puberty. The majority of growth will be completed for girls at the age of 15 and for boys at the age of 16-17. Growth is assessed using data for weight, length or height, head circumference up until age 3, weight for length and Body Mass Index after age 2. Data is plotted on growth charts from the Centers for Disease Control and Prevention (CDC) (or the World Health Organization (WHO) for those up to 2 years of age). Growth is observed over a period of time because a single point is difficult to fully evaluate.

Clinical Significance of CDC Growth Charts

Possible clinical significance is as follows:

- Weight at 50% for age: used as the standard weight for age and sex
- Weight less than10% or greater than 90% for age: may be indicative of the child being underweight or over weight and should be monitored.
- Weight for length at the 50%: Weight is appropriately proportioned for height. As the deviation from the 50% standard becomes greater, growth needs to be fully evaluated for over or under nutrition.
- Length less than10% for age: Length between the 5-10% should be fully evaluated to include changes in growth velocity over time to determine if stunting is acute or chronic. Length less than 5% for age indicates a severe deficit and warrants a full assessment.
- Head circumference less than 5% for age: this can indicate possible chronic malnutrition in-utero or in early infancy.

Marasmus and Kwashiorkor

Marasmus is protein energy malnutrition characterized by depletion in body fat (somatic stores) and muscle mass while visceral protein stores are not affected. Emaciation is common. Children with marasmus may exhibit low body temperature as an adaptive mechanism. Growth is compromised. Kwashiorkor is protein malnutrition characterized by depletion of visceral protein stores while somatic stores and body fat are unaffected. Symptoms of continued protein deprivation are growth failure, edema, poor immunity and reduced muscle mass. Apathy and irritability are seen as well as dermatitis and changes in hair. A common feature of kwashiorkor is a large belly.

Dysphagia

Dysphagia is defined as impaired or difficulty swallowing. Dysphagia can lead to malnutrition because it interferes with the ability to maintain proper nutrition.

Weight loss is common. A speech pathologist should perform an evaluation of swallow function in order to identify ways to help improve the nutritional status of the patient and to prevent medical complications such as aspiration pneumonia or sepsis. The speech pathologist in conjunction with the RD can recommend modifications in texture and/or liquids to assist swallow function along with strategies for increasing acceptance of a texture modified diet such as with spices or presentation. A nasogastric tube may be required to provide short-term nutrition management. A percutaneous endoscopic gastrostomy (PEG) or a gastrostomy-jejunostomy tube may be needed for more permanent management. The overall goal is to prevent malnutrition and improve overall nutritional status.

Professional Practice

Joint Commission on the Accreditation of Healthcare Organizations

The JCAHO is an organization responsible for reviewing standards of care on a voluntary basis to healthcare organizations including hospitals. If an institution desires accreditation with JCAHO, there are many initiatives that must be implemented to help prevent potential errors and improve patient outcomes in all areas of healthcare. If accreditation is received, it means that the institution meets the high standards of care set by the JCAHO. One essential requirement that JCAHO has implemented in 1996 is the reporting of sentinel events. A sentinel event is defined by the JCAHO as an "unexpected occurrence involving death or serious physical or psychological injury or risk thereof." There are many situations that would qualify as sentinel events including medication errors, issues during surgery such as operating on the wrong body part, or hospital acquired infection causing death. The JCAHO collects this information and shares these events across the country along with steps for prevention.

National Quality Forum

The National Quality Forum (NQF) is a compilation of representatives from both the public and private sector. Members include healthcare workers, labor unions, consumers, healthcare institutions, insurance companies, etc. The main goal of this group is improving outcomes of all patients and a national reporting system. This group has over 300 projects including the prevention of malnutrition, controlling infection rates due to central lines, care provided in End Stage Renal Disease, and standards for Adult Diabetes Care. These guidelines are used in healthcare institutions.

Private Insurance Coverage for Patients Receiving Home Nutrition

Insurance coverage for home PN and EN varies widely between insurance companies as well as between contracts. This needs to be fully investigated prior to the start of home therapy. Typically, this is done by the discharge planner or case manager or by the team working with the home care company. For EN, some private insurance companies provide benefits that cover all aspects of home therapy while others cover only the supplies but not the formula. Some provide no coverage at all and the patient would be responsible for paying for enteral therapy. If the patient is responsible for paying for the formula, arrangements must be made for delivery and payment. If patients are not able to afford the cost of enteral formulas, other resources such as a non-profit organization should be investigated. For home PN, prior authorization often needs to be obtained which can sometimes be a lengthy process.

Medicare and Medicare Part B

Medicare is a federal program that provides insurance coverage for people older than 65 or for those that have been disabled for more than 2years. Medicare Part B is a supplemental program that a patient needs to apply for and if accepted, pay out of pocket for. Medicare Part B is the portion that covers home PN and EN. To meet the criteria for coverage, the physician must certify that the patient requires home PN or EN for greater than 90 days. To qualify for home PN, the patient must have tried all other options for nutrition and health maintenance if possible, including diet and tube feeding. Conditions that generally qualify for Medicare Part B coverage include malabsorption, bowel obstruction, certain small bowel fistulas, and pancreatitis. For enteral nutrition to be covered, there must be a functional reason for the patient to be unable to taker oral nutrition, not just because of a poor appetite or weight loss. Reasons can include esophageal obstruction or swallow dysfunction related to stroke.

Therapeutic Plan of Care

Indications for IV Fluids

The indications for the IV fluids are as follows:

- 0.45% NaCl- this is a hypotonic solution called half normal saline used to provide sodium and water. This fluid does not contain dextrose, has 77 mEq/L of sodium and the osmolarity is 154 mOsm/L.
- 0.9% NaCl- this is an isotonic fluid called normal saline for providing extracellular fluid. This fluid does not contain any dextrose, contains 154 mEq/L of sodium and an osmolarity of 308 mOsm/L.
- Lactated Ringers- this is an isotonic solution used for extracellular volume replacement especially around the time of surgery. This fluid does not contain dextrose, has 130 mEq/L of sodium with an osmolarity of 272 mOsm/L. This fluid also contains lactate, potassium and calcium.
- D5W- this is an isotonic solution, which provides water and dextrose for hydration. This fluid contains 50 grams dextrose per liter, is sodium free, and the osmolarity is 250 mOsm/L.
- D5 ½ NS- this is a hypertonic fluid for maintaining or repleting hydration. This fluid contains 50 grams dextrose per liter, 77 mEq/L sodium and the osmolarity is 405 mOsm/L.
- D10W- this is a hypertonic fluid used for hydration. This fluid contains 100 grams pf dextrose per liter, is sodium free and has an osmolarity of 500 mOsm/L.

Calculating Fluid Requirements for Children

Using the Holliday-Segar Method for assessing fluid requirements, maintenance fluid for a child 0-10 kg will be 100 ml/kg, for a child 10-20 kg will be 1000 ml + 50 ml/kg above 10 kg, and for weight greater than 20 kg, fluid requirements will be 1500 ml + 20 ml/kg for weight over 20 kg. Fluid intake may need to be adjusted based on insensible or sensible losses. Children with special healthcare needs may not be able to indicate thirst on their own or may not be able to physically take a drink themselves. Excessive drooling may be an issue. Physical activity may be limited or absent which in turn can affect bowel function and cause increased fluid loss through diarrhea. Diarrhea can also occur with certain medications. Children with a neurogenic bladder need to be sure they receive enough fluid and that the bladder is emptied often to prevent bladder infections. Children with Down Syndrome sometimes have cardiac defects that may require fluid restriction.

Indirect Calorimetry in Assessing Energy Requirements in ICU Patients

Indirect calorimetry is a way to assess energy requirements that measures oxygen consumption and carbon dioxide production. It is generally the best and most accurate way to measure resting energy expenditure (REE) in ICU patients. IC is a useful tool to determine if appropriate nutrition support is being provided to a patient especially where there are indicators that would suggest otherwise such as poor wound healing or inability to wean from the ventilator. A metabolic cart is required. Factors that affect the accuracy of IC include the presence of an air leak, patients who are not receiving a continuous form of nutrition (i.e. intermittent tube feedings or cyclic TPN), or hemodialysis within 4 hours of the study. Other factors that can affect the results are nursing care provided during the study which interrupts the steady state or mechanical ventilator settings of FiO2 greater than 60 or positive end expiratory pressure (PEEP) greater than12 cm H2O. The inability to achieve steady state where whole body oxygen (VO2) and carbon dioxide (VCO2) do not vary more than 10% will also affect results.

Interpreting Resting Energy Expenditure and Respiratory Quotient

Before the REE and RQ are interpreted, the IC study should be reviewed to make sure the results are valid and a steady state was achieved. In the past, an activity factor of 5-10% was added to the REE to cover any physical activity incurred in the ICU setting. Current practice is to provide patients with only the REE without the additional factors. Total calories are provided, not non-protein calories. The RQ is the ratio of carbon dioxide produced to oxygen consumed. It provides an idea of what type of substrate is being utilized. An RQ less than 0.82 may mean the patient is not receiving sufficient calories and is burning fat stores. An RQ of 0.85 indicates mixed fuel (carbohydrate, protein, fat) and indicates the patient is being fed at the appropriate energy level. An RQ greater than 1.0 indicates the patient is receiving too many calories, which can lead to fat deposition and increased work of breathing.

Calculating Energy Requirements Using kcal/kg

Utilizing a simple equation for estimating energy requirements is well accepted by many dietetic practitioners. This is a range of 20-35 kcal/kg for the adult population with an initial goal of 25 kcal/kg. This plan should be continually evaluated and the caloric goals adjusted according to medical status.

Overfeeding

Overfeeding a patient can be dangerous because it can increase carbon dioxide production thus interfering with weaning from the ventilator. Overfeeding can cause elevated blood glucose levels, elevated triglycerides, and changes in fluid balance.

Underfeeding

Underfeeding a patient who is critically ill can cause weight loss or loss of lean body mass, can delay wound healing and can lead to nosocomial infections. Underfeeding may also prevent weaning from the ventilator because of respiratory muscle weakness. Underfeeding may impair immune function and may also alter organ function.

Harris Benedict Method

The Harris Benedict Method for estimating calorie requirements was published in 1919 and predicts the basal metabolic rate for men and women.

The equation to estimate energy requirements:

- for men= 66 + 13.75(wt in kg) + 5(ht in cm) – 6.8(age in years)
- for women= 655 + 9.6(wt in kg) + 1.8(ht in cm) – 4.7(age in years)

Additional percentages are added on to the result to account for activity and stress for disease. Factors that may affect the accuracy of the predictive equation is that the data was collected over 90 years ago and does not reflect the current population in terms of race, weight or differences in body size. Many clinicians use an adjusted body weight in the equation instead of actual body weight. This is not the intent of this method and by using an adjusted body weight, energy requirements may be underestimated especially for those with obesity.

Effect on Protein Requirements by Critical Illness

In critical illness, the patient is at risk for losing lean body mass because protein needs are elevated. The body will use its own stores of protein to meet demands if insufficient protein is provided. In metabolic stress, the body needs amino acids for gluconeogenesis and needs to produce acute phase proteins such as C Reactive protein. It also tries to maintain immune function to prevent infection, to heal wounds and is required by the kidney to maintain acid base balance. Providing sufficient protein to prevent catabolism and loss of lean body tissue is extremely important. Patients who may require greater than1.5 grams protein/kg are patients receiving CVVHD (continuous veno-venous hemodialysis), some patients with cirrhosis, short bowel syndrome/malabsorption, burns, large wounds, and in the immediate post operative period for organ transplants.

Carbohydrate Requirements for Adults and Children

Carbohydrate requirements are estimated to be approximately 45-60% of total calories. For infants, the requirements range from 30-60% of total calories. Adults need a minimum of 50 grams of carbohydrate per day to prevent ketosis. Adults have approximately 200 grams of carbohydrate in storage available for ready use. If blood glucose levels drop, the liver will release its glycogen stores although these stores are limited. The body will then synthesize glucose from non-carbohydrate sources such as amino acids and fatty acids (gluconeogenesis). As the fasting period continues, the body begins to adapt by using less glucose. The body produces less insulin and more glucagon. Rates of fatty acid oxidation increase and the main source of energy is from fat stores. Ketone bodies are produced and used as fuel by the heart and skeletal muscles. The metabolic rate is lowered. After 1-2 weeks, the brain adapts to fasting and will begin to use ketones for energy as well. The use of ketone bodies for energy preserves lean body mass.

Medium Chain Triglycercides

Medium chain triglycerides (MCT) are saturated fatty acids with a carbon length of 6-12 chains. They are soluble in water and do not require bile acids or pancreatic lipase for absorption. MCT enter the liver through the portal vein as free fatty acids. MCT are digested quickly and are used as a caloric source. MCT is not stored in adipose tissue. Patients with fat malabsorption due to pancreatic insufficiency or resection of the intestines may benefit from the use of MCT. Patients with bile acid insufficiency or defects in the lymphatic system would also benefit.

Short Chain Fatty Acids

Short chain fatty acids (SCFA) are fatty acids with 4-6 carbon length. Some SCFA are found in foods such as butter or dairy products. The main source in the body is from the fermentation of non-digestible carbohydrates and fiber that occurs in the large intestine. Bacteria in the colon are responsible for this process. SCFA are quickly absorbed by the mucosa in the intestines and colon. The benefits of SCFA are as a main source of food for colonocytes, the assistance with water and sodium regulation, and the contribution to the overall health of the intestinal mucosa. In the long term, SCFA are believed to help prevent diseases of the intestine such as cancer. Research into this area continues in the use of SCFA and intestinal adaptation in patients with short gut.

Enteral and Parenteral Requirements for Iron

Dietary Reference Intakes for iron from the Food and Nutrition Board of the Institute of Medicine are as follows: 0-6 months 0.27 mg, 7-12 months 11 mg, 1-3 years 7 mg, 4-8 years 10 mg and 9-13 years 8 mg. For males 14-18 years, requirements are 11 mg and older than 18 years 8 mg. For females 14-18 years, requirements are 15 mg, 18-50 years 18 mg, and older than 50 years requirements are 8 mg. In pregnancy, requirements increase to 27 mg and lactation 9- 10 mg depending on age of mother. The recommendation for parenteral iron for adults is 150-200 mg of elemental iron per day.

For children, the amount of parenteral iron needed can be calculated using the following equation:

- Fe (mg)= wt (kg) x 4.5 x (13.5- patients hemoglobin [g/dl])

There are three forms of parenteral iron. Sodium ferric acid and iron sucrose are the first two forms. These forms have a lower risk for the occurrence of side effects. The third form is iron dextran, which has been associated with side effects including anaphylactic reactions. Iron dextran is the type of iron supplement used in parenteral nutrition solutions. A test dose of iron dextran must be given before a full dose is administered.

Enteral and Parenteral Requirements for Adult Males (Age 51-70 Years)

For enteral requirements using the Dietary Reference Intakes from the Food and Nutrition Board of the Institute of Medicine are:

- Zinc 11 mg/day
- Copper 900 mcg/day
- Chromium 30 mcg/day
- Manganese 2.3 mg/day
- Selenium 55 mcg/day

For daily parenteral requirements according to the American Society for Parenteral and Enteral Nutrition (ASPEN, 2004) are:

- Zinc 2.5-5 mg
- Copper 0.3-0.5 mg
- Chromium 10-15 mcg
- Manganese 60-100 mcg
- Selenium 20-60 mg

Additional zinc, copper, and chromium should be provided if the patient is experiencing increased GI losses. Additional zinc should be added for patients who are hypermetabolic. Patients with cholestasis should have copper and manganese omitted because of the risk for toxicity due to decreased excretion. Patients with renal insufficiency or failure should have selenium and chromium omitted due to decreased excretion and risk for toxicity.

Parenteral Vitamins and Minerals Requirements

Parenteral vitamins and minerals do not need to go through digestion and absorption to be utilized thus parenteral requirements are lower than the Dietary Reference Intakes (DRI). The Food and Drug Administration (FDA) reevaluated dosing requirements in 2000. Daily requirements are as follows: vitamin A 1 mg, vitamin D 5 mcg, vitamin E 10 mg, vitamin K 150 mcg, thiamin 3 mg, riboflavin 3.6 mg, vitamin B6 6 mg, vitamin B12 5 mcg, niacin 40 mg, folic acid 600 mcg, pantothenic acid 15 mg, biotin 60 mcg, vitamin C 200 mg. Daily requirements for parenteral calcium are 10-15 mEq, magnesium 8-20 mEq and phosphate 20-40 mmol. Daily requirements for sodium range from 1-2 mEq/kg and potassium 1-2 mEq/kg. Acetate and chloride are provided as needed to keep acid base balance within normal range.

Calculating Insulin Requirements for Tube Feeding

If IV insulin is not an option, subcutaneous insulin will need to be given. The patient's basal insulin requirements as well as the amount of insulin needed to cover carbohydrate intake will need to be calculated. The average requirement is 1 unit of insulin for each 10 grams of carbohydrate. Requirements will vary depending upon the patient's weight, presence of abdominal obesity, use of corticosteroids and sensitivity to insulin. Insulin doses from the patient's home regimen are also useful in calculating insulin requirements while receiving tube feedings. A combination of regular and intermediate acting insulin given every 6 hours can be effective in controlling BG levels for patients receiving continuous tube feedings. Long acting insulin given every 24 hours with regular insulin given every 6 hours or a combination of regular and intermediate given every 12 hours is also a possibility. Short or rapid acting insulin can be supplemented as needed. For patients receiving bolus tube feedings, rapid acting insulin can be used. The main goal is normoglycemia.

Short Bowel Syndrome

Short Bowel Syndrome (SBS) occurs following a major intestinal resection. A patient is considered to have SBS if the length of small bowel is 100-120 cm without a colon or 50 cm or less with a colon. Patients with less than 100 cm of small bowel remaining without a colon will likely require a lifetime of parenteral nutrition (PN). Complications of SBS are significant and potentially life threatening and can include weight loss, malnutrition, issues with fluid and electrolyte management and malabsorption of fat-soluble vitamins and vitamin B12. Bile salt malabsorption and resultant fat malabsorption can be complications of an ileal resection. The gut does have the ability to adapt and this process can take a couple years. Factors that influence bowel adaptation are length of the remaining jejunum and ileum, presence of the colon and presence of the ileocecal valve. The age of the patient, nutritional status and the introduction of enteral nutrition also play a role in adaptation.

Medications Used to Manage Short Bowel Syndrome

Medications commonly used in the management of SBS include:

- Histamine receptor antagonists (H2 blockers) and proton inhibitors – prescribed to control excessive gastric acid production and regulate pH level.
- Octreotide- sometimes prescribed for patients with increased stoma output or diarrhea to help reduce pancreatic and gastric secretions.
- Antidiarrheal medications- prescribed to control stool output and slow transit time especially for patients who have had an ileal or colon resection or patients without an ileocecal valve.
- Cholestyramine- sometimes prescribed for patients with diarrhea or steatorrhea to bind bile salts especially those who have had significant ileal resection.
- Antibiotics- often prescribed for patients at risk for developing bacterial overgrowth in the small bowel. Patients without an ileocecal valve and with reduced gastric acid production are at risk.

Oral Diet Modifications Recommended for Patients with Short Bowel Syndrome

Enteral nutrition (oral or tube feedings) should begin as soon as possible to begin the adaptation process. For patients with a colon, 50-60% of total calories should be from carbohydrates, 20-30% from protein and 20-30% from fat. For patients with a jejunostomy or ileostomy, carbohydrate intake should be 20-30% of total calories and 50-60% from fat. Patients with SBS require significantly higher amounts of calories to account for malabsorption (up to 400% of their normal requirements). Simple sugars should be avoided because this can cause osmotic diarrhea. The higher amounts of complex carbohydrate and fiber rich foods in the diet will allow the carbohydrate to be converted to short chain fatty acids through the fermentation of bacteria in the colon and used as energy. Small, frequent meals and snacks are recommended. Fluids should be taken separately from meals to help reduce gastric emptying. Oxalate containing foods may need to be restricted to prevent oxalate kidney stones.

Body Mass Index Range for Normal Weight, Overweight, and Class I, II, and III Obesity

The BMI range for normal weight is 18.5-24.9 kg/m^2, for overweight 25.0-29.0 kg/m^2, for Class I obesity 30.0-34.9 kg/m^2, for Class II obesity 35.0-39.9 kg/m^2, and for Class III obesity 40 kg/m^2 or greater. The BMI is a useful tool for assessing morbidity and mortality. The higher the BMI value, the higher the risk for developing co-morbidities and/or death. These co-morbidities include heart disease, pulmonary disease including obstructive sleep apnea and hypoventilation syndrome, gastroesophageal reflux, Type 2 Diabetes Mellitus, cellulitus and poor wound healing, and various types of cancers. Higher BMI's are also associated with arthritis and back problems. Social issues are also an issue and include discrimination and reduced quality of life. Fat that is located around the abdominal area (called "apple" shape) increases the risk for diabetes, elevated lipids, heart disease and high blood pressure. Abdominal fat is also a factor for the metabolic syndrome.

Candidates for Bariatric Surgery and the Laparoscopic Adjustable Gastric Band

Patients who are potential candidates for bariatric surgery should have a BMI greater than 40 kg/m^2 or a BMI greater than 35 kg/m^2 with additional co-morbidities such as hypertension or heart disease. All candidates should also have made concerted attempts at weight loss including medically supervised calorie controlled diets. The Laparoscopic Adjustable Gastric Band (LAGB) is the easiest procedure to complete and can be reversed if needed. The procedure involves the placement of a band between the gastroesophageal junction and the upper part of the stomach to form a smaller reservoir. Over time, the pouch will hold approximately 4-5 ounces. The length of hospital stay is short and patients return to normal activity quickly. Complications can include slippage of the band, enlargement of the pouch, or wearing away of the band. If complications are present, the patient may experience vomiting or fail to lose weight. Other side effects can be reflux. Successful weight loss can be 30% or more of their pre-surgical weight.

Gastric Bypass

Gastric bypass surgery involves surgically reducing the size of the stomach. This is considered a major surgical procedure and can be done open or laparoscopically. The smaller pouch is created and divided from the remainder of the stomach and is then reattached at a lower point in the small intestine. The size of the new pouch is initially about 1 ounce but over time will stretch to 4-8 ounce capacity. The hospital stay is longer and recuperation takes approximately 2 weeks. Patients can experience dumping syndrome and intolerance to high fat foods. Patients who overeat and fail to follow the appropriate diet may experience vomiting, weight loss failure or rupture of the pouch. There is a possibility of iron, vitamin B12 or folate deficiency. Patients may also develop gastritis, reflux, gallstones or ventral hernias following the procedure. Successful weight loss can be 60% or more of the original excess weight.

Nutrient Deficiencies Following a Total Gastrectomy

Pernicious anemia (vitamin B12 deficiency) can occur because of the lack of intrinsic factor needed to facilitate the absorption of vitamin B12 in the ileum. Folate deficiency can also occur most likely due to malabsorption. Iron deficiency is common. Possible causes for this include decreased gastric acid, which is required to convert iron into the ferrous form for better absorption. Poor dietary iron intake is a possibility. In addition, the duodenum, which is the main site for iron absorption, is usually bypassed during the resection. Bone disease such as osteoporosis, osteomalacia or osteopenia is a complication seen following a total gastrectomy and its causes are multifactorial. Reduced intakes of calcium and vitamin D are common. Lactose if often avoided because lactose intolerance can develop following a total gastrectomy. The avoidance of lactose containing foods also limits calcium and vitamin D intake. Metabolism of calcium and vitamin D is altered and the 25- dihydroxy vitamin D level should be monitored.

Dumping Syndrome

Dumping syndrome can occur following a gastrectomy because normal GI regulation is lost. Stomach contents move quickly into the small intestine producing a hyperosmolar load. Symptoms can range from diarrhea as a result of the hyperosmolar load to abdominal cramping and fullness to vomiting. A patient may experience weakness, flushing or sweating following a meal. In patients who have also had a vagotomy, diarrhea may increase in incidence after consuming fluids with meals. Small, frequent meals are recommended. Patients should sit upright while eating and chew food well. Fluids should be limited or avoided at meals. High sugar foods and beverages can also cause symptoms of dumping syndrome and should be avoided. A protein source should be consumed at each meal and snack. Selection of high fiber foods is important as this will help to slow transit time and promote nutrient absorption.

Nutrient Absorption in the Duodenum, Jejunum, Ileum and Colon

The small intestine is made up of three sections- the duodenum, jejunum, and ileum. The duodenum is the main site for absorption of iron, folate, calcium, magnesium and zinc. The jejunum is the main site for absorption of glucose, galactose, fructose and water-soluble vitamins. The ileum is the main site of absorption for amino acids, dipeptides, fat-soluble vitamins and cholesterol. The terminal ileum is responsible for the absorption of bile salts and vitamin B12. The colon, also known as the large intestine, is where sodium, potassium and water are absorbed. The ileocecal valve is located between the ileum and the cecum and acts to control the passage of digestive material into the colon.

Crohn's Disease and Ulcerative Colitis

Inflammatory Bowel Disease (IBD) is generally diagnosed in patients aged 15-30 years although it can occur later in life as well. The two main forms of IBD are Crohn's disease and Ulcerative Colitis. The causes of IBD are still undetermined. Crohn's disease, also known as regional enteritis, most commonly involves the distal ileum and colon but any part of the GI tract can be affected. The disease can occur in different parts of the intestine. Diagnosis is determined by identification of clinical symptoms, and endoscopic and biopsy evaluation. Diarrhea is common. Anal abscesses and fistulas are commonly seen. Surgery is required in 50-75% of cases but is not curative and can result in malabsorption. Ulcerative Colitis (UC) is found only in the colon and it involves a continuous disease process unlike Crohn's disease. The majority of UC cases have rectal involvement. Diarrhea and rectal bleeding are usually present. In severe cases, the colon is removed and an ileostomy is created. Both forms of IBD can experience weight loss, malnutrition, and food intolerances, and can develop a fear of eating relating to exacerbation of symptoms.

Nutritional Management of Crohn's Disease

In Crohn's disease, calorie requirements are not usually elevated. Protein needs may range from 1-1.5 gm/kg depending upon protein losses related to inflammation. The main theory regarding diet therapy for Crohn's disease is that of individual tolerance. Patients with strictures will need to follow a low fiber diet but studies have not shown that a long term diet low in fiber for other patients with Crohn's disease to be beneficial or improve the course of the disease. Lactose should be avoided if a lactose deficiency is present. The use of enteral nutrition is successful in pediatric patients with Crohn's disease to reverse growth failure. Corticosteroids are still the most effective therapy. No single enteral formulation (elemental, semi elemental or polymeric) has been shown to be completely effective. Parenteral nutrition should not be the primary mode of therapy in Crohn's disease unless there is a contraindication to oral or enteral nutrition. Common nutrient deficiencies can include iron, calcium, vitamin D, and possibly vitamin K and should be supplemented accordingly.

Medical Nutrition Therapy for a Patient with an Enterocutaneous Fistula

An enterocutaneous (EC) fistula is an abnormal opening involving the skin and the intestines. EC fistulas can occur following bowel resection, pancreatic surgery, lysis of adhesions, or after surgery is performed emergently in the bowel without time to prep the bowel first. Fistulas can also occur in conditions relating to the GI tract such as IBD, bowel ischemia or perforation, cancer, radiation therapy or abdominal trauma. Parenteral nutrition (PN) has historically been used as the primary mode of nutrition support for patients with EC fistulas. Enteral feedings have been successfully trialed and can be considered when planning nutritional care.

Favorable factors for providing enteral nutrition include:

- Fistula output less than 500 ml per day
- Fistula location in the distal ileum or colon
- Fistula in the esophagus, duodenum or proximal jejunum where enteral nutrition can be provided distal to the fistula

Enteral Formulas Appropriate for Use in a Patient with an Enterocutaneous Fistula

The type of formula used will vary depending upon the patient. For patients with a distal fistula, a low fiber formula should be used to reduce fistula output. An elemental or semi elemental formula can be used for patients losing pancreatic and biliary secretions that are not reinfused back in to the body. This may help with digestion and absorption. Some patients may require supplemental IV fluids to assist with maintaining hydration and electrolytes. Patients with high output fistulas in the jejunum or ileum, a pancreatic fistula or a fistula where the drainage cannot be controlled and prevented from coming in contact with skin will require bowel rest and parenteral nutrition.

Enteral Nutrition in Ileus, Partial Small Bowel Obstruction, Vomiting, and Diarrhea

A patient with an ileus or a partial small bowel obstruction does not always preclude the use of enteral nutrition. Often times the feeding tube can be successfully placed in the small bowel below the ileus or the obstruction. Studies have shown that the lack of bowel sounds does not necessarily preclude enteral nutrition. For patients experiencing vomiting, a feeding tube placed in the small bowel coupled with a tube for gastric decompression has been tried with success. For patients with diarrhea, the cause and type should be determined. However, for patients with intractable vomiting and diarrhea that is not responsive to medical intervention will likely need parenteral nutrition.

Protein and Calorie Requirements for Patients with Cirrhosis

The majority of patients who have stable liver disease can tolerate normal amounts of protein without adverse effects. Calorie levels are also provided at usual requirements. For patients with cirrhosis but without encephalopathy, a protein restriction is not required. A protein goal of 1-1.2 gm/kg is reasonable. If malnutrition is present, protein intake may need to increase up to 2 gm/kg. Calorie requirements are estimated at 25-35 kcal/kg and up to 40 kcal/kg with malnutrition. For patients with cirrhosis and acute hepatic encephalopathy (HE), protein should be restricted to 0.6-0.8 gm/kg until symptoms of HE clears. Protein intake should then increase to 1-1.2 gm/kg. Calorie requirements are estimated at 35 kcal/kg to help spare protein. For patients with cirrhosis and chronic HE, a protein restriction of 0.6-0.8 gm/kg is recommended. Symptoms of chronic HE does not generally clear and the patient's mental status is chronically impaired. These patients may require 30-40 kcal/kg. The use of branch chain amino acids (BCAA) as a treatment for HE has not been proven to be effective and formulas containing BCAA are very costly.

Chronic Pancreatitis

Chronic pancreatitis is a chronic inflammation of the pancreas that leads to irreversible damage to the endocrine and exocrine function of the pancreas. Alcohol abuse is the most common cause. Symptoms of chronic pancreatitis are the same as acute pancreatitis. The nutritional management of chronic pancreatitis first involves avoiding alcohol. If alcohol is avoided, symptoms may abate and the patient may be able to eat more on his own to improve nutritional status. The patient should consume approximately 35 kcal/kg with 1-1.5 gm/kg of protein. Fat intake should be reduced to help decrease pancreatic enzyme secretion. The use of MCT oil may also decrease pancreatic stimulation and allow for weight gain. Some patients require pancreatic enzyme replacement therapy to treat steatorrhea. Enzyme supplements will also help with pain control and enable the patient to consume better nutrition. For severe cases that are not responsive to an oral diet, a nasojejunal tube or more permanent enteral access may be required. Parenteral nutrition is used as a last step for patients without enteral access.

Acute Pancreatitis

Acute pancreatitis is a hypermetabolic process that increases energy requirements approximately 40% above those calculated using the Harris Benedict equation. The stress of acute pancreatitis can lead to muscle breakdown and an increase in oxidative stress. Acute pancreatitis will impair a patient's ability to eat due to nausea, vomiting and abdominal pain. Hyperglycemia and fat malabsorption are possible complications. Historically, pancreatic rest and parenteral nutrition (PN) was believed to be the most effective treatment of acute pancreatitis. Studies have demonstrated that enteral nutrition is now preferred over PN. Enteral nutrition helps preserve gut integrity. An isotonic 1 kcal/ml formula is the formula of choice and should be initiated within 72 hours of admission. A nasojejunal tube should be placed and the tip should be located past the Ligament of Treitz. For symptoms of intolerance such as an increase in amylase or lipase levels, fever or an increase in WBC, diarrhea or abdominal pain, an elemental very low fat formula or a semi elemental formula containing MCT should be tried before PN is initiated.

Chronic Kidney Disease

CDK is permanent damage to the kidneys. This can occur because of a disease such as diabetes mellitus or as a result of physical damage to the kidney. There is a resultant decrease in the glomerular filtration rate (GFR), decrease in the kidney's ability to excrete waste and produce urine, and regulate electrolytes. The goal of treatment is to preserve as much kidney function as possible. Patients who develop CKD are at risk for malnutrition. Calorie requirements are estimated to be 30-40 kcal/kg per day although additional co-morbidities such as respiratory failure or sepsis may further increase calorie requirements. Protein requirements for CDK are 0.6-0.8 gm/kg per day, which are designed to help control uremia and to hold off on the need for dialysis as long as possible.

Dialysis

Hemodialysis is one type of dialysis that involves the circulation of blood outside the body into filters that remove waste products a few times per week. CAPD is a second type of dialysis that involves the use of a dialysate and the body's peritoneal membrane to remove waste. The third type is continuous renal replacement therapy that involves utilizing hemodialysis for 24 hours per day. Once hemodialysis or CAPD is started, protein requirements will increase to 1.2-1.3

gm/kg per day. Patients receiving continuous renal replacement therapy may require up to 2.5 gm/kg per day. For patients receiving CAPD, up to 75% of the dextrose form the dialysate can be absorbed by the body and used as a calorie source because of the length of the dwell times. These calories will need to be taken into account when estimating energy requirements.

Protein and Calorie Requirements in Patients with Pulmonary Disease

Indirect calorimetry is the preferred method for assessing energy requirements for patients with pulmonary failure. The respiratory quotient (RQ) should be monitored. Care should be given not to overfeed which can impede ventilator weaning. If indirect calorimetry is not available, 25-30 kcal/kg can be provided. Actual body weight should be used for the calculation for patients below their ideal body weight (IBW) up to 24% above their IBW to help prevent overfeeding. For patients who are 25% or more above their ideal body weight, an adjusted body weight can be used.

This can be calculated using the following equation:

- Adjusted Body Weight= [(actual body weight- IBW) x 0.25] + IBW

Protein requirements are estimated to be approximately 1.2-1.5 grams/kg using the lower of the two weights (actual or ideal).

Effects of Nutritional Status on Pulmonary Disease

Patients with pulmonary failure are at risk for protein calorie malnutrition. These patients exert a substantial amount of energy just to breathe. Weight loss is common due to this increased work of breathing. Many patients lose weight during an acute flare, however, fail to regain the weight when the disease is better managed. Baseline anthropometrics are useful to monitor weight changes. Patients with pulmonary failure are also at risk for loss of lean body mass. Inadequate calorie and protein intake can lead to a loss of respiratory muscles including the diaphragm, which will further impact breathing. Many patients with malnutrition will have hypoalbuminemia that can lead to pulmonary edema and further complicate the pulmonary disease. Malnutrition also affects immune function, which can lead to lung infections. Hypophosphatemia is also a possibility with malnutrition especially during refeeding. Low serum phosphorus will impair oxygen delivery.

Nutrition Care Plan for a Patient with a Stage III Non-Healing Pressure Ulcer

Pressure ulcers are usually classified in 4 stages.

- Stage I- redness or other superficial, minor changes in skin integrity which will usually heal on their own when pressure on the area is relieved
- Stage II- superficial changes in skin that appear as a blister or minor ulceration. These ulcers will heal without issue if treatment is initiated without delay.

- Stage III- the pressure ulcer has extended down below the skin and the wound appears deep
- Stage IV- these are generally the most serious and the wound can extend deeply into the muscle and bone. Because these wounds are large and deep, the patient is at risk for infection. These sores are the most difficult to heal.

The most common cause of pressure sores is failure to change positions often. This can be due to paralysis or immobilization. The patients most at risk for pressure sores are the elderly, patients in nursing homes, presence of malnutrition or reduced fat stores, presence of incontinence or patients with low or no pain tolerance.

Without any conditions that would adversely affect recommendations, the patient would ideally require approximately 30 kcal/kg with 1.25- 1.5 grams/kg of protein per day. Fluid requirements would be 30-35 cc/kg. Vitamin and mineral supplementation is essential to wound healing. In addition to a multivitamin and mineral complex, vitamin C should be supplemented up to 2000 mg per day and zinc should be supplemented at 25-30 mg of elemental zinc. Zinc is normally provided as zinc sulfate and the standard dose of 220 mg of zinc sulfate provides 50 mg elemental zinc. Additional vitamin A can be supplemented if needed.

Traumatic Brain Injury

The body's response to a TBI is a significantly increased metabolic state. Production of negative acute phase reactants such as albumin and prealbumin are decreased while production of positive acute phase reactants such as C reactive protein, cortisol, and growth hormone are increased in response to this metabolic stress. Protein catabolism is significant and usually reaches its peak by 2 weeks. Fluid balance is of utmost importance to prevent cerebral edema. Providing too much free water to patients following TBI can seriously alter sodium balance. Mannitol is often used as an osmotic diuretic, which also makes balancing fluid and electrolytes a challenge. Hyperglycemia should be prevented because blood glucose levels greater than 220 mg/dl are associated with unfavorable neurological recovery. Indirect calorimetry is the preferred method for assessing energy requirements. If this is not feasible, the Brain Trauma Foundation recommends using 40% above the basal energy requirements calculated using the Harris Benedict equation. Protein requirements are 1.5-2 grams/kg with close monitoring of renal function.

Enteral Nutrition in Patients with Traumatic Brain Injury

Patients with TBI are often placed on mechanical ventilation following the initial injury. Enteral nutrition is the preferred feeding modality. Nasoduodenal or nasojejunal tubes can help to decrease rates of aspiration and feeding intolerance commonly seen in patients with TBI. These types of tubes may increase intracranial pressure and would not be indicated in this scenario. A gastrojejunostomy tube placed percutaneously is another option. Early nutrition within 48 hours is an important step to help slow catabolism, prevent weight loss, reduce the inflammatory response, protect immune function and encourage favorable neurological outcome. Low rate tube feedings in conjunction with parenteral nutrition is an option for patients who do not tolerate full enteral nutrition. This use of trophic feeding stimulates gut function and helps to prevent bacterial translocation.

Nutritional Care of the Patient with Spinal Cord Injury in the Acute Stage

Patients with acute Spinal Cord Injury generally have lower calorie requirements than would be predicted using the Harrison Benedict equation and adding a stress factor. Calorie requirements could be reduced up to 90% of basal energy requirements (BEE). In general, the higher the injury is on the spinal cord, the lower the calorie requirements. Paraplegic patients may require approximately 28 kcal/kg while quadriplegic patients may need only approximately 23 kcal/kg. Protein requirements, however, are elevated in part to the use of high dose steroids. Nutrition support should be started within 72 hours of admission following acute injury. Nasogastric or nasojejunal tubes may be the best choice to help prevent complications such as high gastric residuals. Metoclopramide is contraindicated in patients with Spinal Cord Injury related to possible side effects such as muscle spasms. Fluid status should be monitored closely as hyponatremia can easily occur with too much free water.

Nutritional Care of the Patient with Spinal Cord Injury in the Rehabilitative Stage

When the patient with a Spinal Cord Injury is stable enough to move into rehabilitation, energy requirements may be further reduced and should be frequently reassessed, as the potential for obesity is a concern. Protein losses may continue due to muscle catabolism related to immobility. With aggressive physical therapy and adequate protein intake, the patient may be able to rebuild some muscle mass. Renal function should be closely monitored as function may gradually decline. Overall nutritional status needs continued monitoring as depression and poor intake can occur and adversely affect nutritional status. Patients with spinal cord injuries are also at risk for pressure sores. An adequate bowel regimen is also recommended.

Tolerance to Gastric and Small Bowel Feedings in Trauma Patients

Enteral nutrition should be started as soon as possible in trauma patients who will not be able to meet nutritional requirements within 3-5 days. A nasogastric tube is often the easiest route for providing enteral nutrition, however, many ICU patients will develop intolerance related to a delay in gastric emptying. This can be due to sepsis, peritonitis, hemodynamic instability, low flow state, or pneumonia. Aspiration remains a risk with nasogastric feeding, however, elevated gastric residuals are not always a seen in patients with aspiration. Small bowel feedings are often better tolerated especially for those patients who have had major abdominal surgery, an aspiration event or for patients who are unable to have the head of the bed elevated or have consistently high gastric residuals. Many medications such as paralyzing agents or sedatives will also have an effect on tolerance.

Sepsis

Sepsis is the systemic response by the body to infection. Systemic Inflammatory Response Syndrome (SIRS) can develop with symptoms of fever, rapid heart rate, rapid respirations and organ dysfunction especially of the heart, lungs, kidney, and liver. During sepsis, protein catabolism occurs at a significant rate resulting in net negative nitrogen balance. Providing adequate protein to a patient with sepsis will help the liver to keep producing acute phase reactant proteins such as C reactive protein but will not stop the catabolic process totally. Without a source of protein, significant amounts of lean body mass will be lost each day. The longer the catabolic period, the greater the protein losses from skeletal muscles, which can adversely affect pulmonary status, immune function and the ability to recuperate.

Metabolic Response During Sepsis

Hyperglycemia and insulin resistance are common during sepsis. Catabolic hormones such as glucagon and cortisol are released by the body in response to stress. This causes glycogenolysis and gluconeogenesis to occur. Glycogen stores are quickly depleted and the body shifts to using lipids and protein as a fuel source. Sepsis also causes cells to take in less glucose. This coupled with an increase in endogenous glucose production causes insulin resistance leading to elevated glucose levels. Other catabolic hormones such as epinephrine and norepinephrine as well as glucagon are produced during sepsis and cause stored triglycerides to break down to glycerol and free fatty acids (lypolysis). Long chain fatty acids are not able to move into the mitochondria. The body's ability to use the Kreb's Cycle for energy production is impaired as well as the process of ketogenesis. This affects the body's ability to use ketoacids as an alternate fuel source. Additionally, lipoprotein lipase activity is also impaired which can lead to hyperlipidemia, hyperglycemia and hyperlactemia.

Consideration for Providing Carbohydrate and Lipids During Sepsis

Carbohydrates should be provided at 50-60% of total calories. The glucose infusion rate should be provided at 4-6 mg/kg/minute. If the glucose oxidative rate is exceeded, hyperglycemia and lipogenesis will occur. Glucose levels should be closely m monitored and kept between 90-110 mg/dl to minimize complications from hyperglycemia and to potentially improve outcome. During sepsis, intravenous fat as soybean oil should be restricted to 1 gram/kg because of the alteration in lipid metabolism that occurs during sepsis. In other parts of the world, lipid formulations that include olive oil, fish oil, or medium chain triglycerides (MCT) are available and are better utilized by the body. The use of fish oil has been extensively studied and the benefits include an improved immune response.

Energy and Protein Requirements During Sepsis

Energy requirements can range from 20-60% above basal energy requirements (BEE) predicted by the Harris Benedict Equation. These requirements can remain elevated for up to 3 weeks following a septic event. However, because of the body's metabolic response to stress, the body will not be able to utilize the energy efficiently, therefore, underfeeding during the initial few days of sepsis may be warranted. A range of 20- 30 kcal/kg is appropriate. Protein requirements are estimated at 1.5-2 grams/kg but may be even higher for patients with burn injury or other large wounds. Specific amino acids such as arginine and glutamine considered conditionally essential during periods of stress are being diligently studied. Arginine, which is believed to help the body's immune response, is added to immune enhanced formulas but data remains conflicted as to the appropriate dosing. Glutamine is used as a fuel source in the gut and studies have shown an overall benefit to its use in reducing length of hospital stay, lower infection rates, and better mortality rates.

Enteral and Parenteral Nutrition for Patients with Cancer

Cancer patients who are not able to eat and are at risk for malnutrition should be evaluated for specialized nutrition support. Patients with cancer of the head and neck will receive benefits from enteral nutrition. These patients often have malnutrition when cancer treatment is starting. Placement of percutaneous endoscopic gastrostomy tubes (PEG) can help prevent dehydration, improve nutritional status, and assist with weight gain if placed prior to or during surgical resection. Patients with other types of cancer may not benefit as well in terms of improved mortality but may have a shorter length of hospital stay and lower chance for complications when enteral nutrition is used. Parenteral nutrition can be an option for malnourished cancer patients actively receiving treatment but who have developed severe GI side effects, which are not expected to resolve within 1-2 weeks.

Effect of Radiation & Chemotherapy Treatments on the Nutritional Status of Patients

Radiation therapy in the oropharyngeal or abdominal area can be a significant factor in developing malnutrition. In the oropharyngeal area, loss of taste, dryness of the mouth and pain with swallowing can occur. Radiation to the neck area can cause dysphagia, esophagitis, and strictures which all limits the patient's ability to eat adequately. Radiation to the abdominal area can cause short or long-term damage to the bowel resulting in diarrhea, malabsorption, bowel obstructions or fistulas. Chemotherapy is used to destroy cancer cells but it also can cause injury to normal cells especially in any part of the gastrointestinal tract. Chemotherapy can cause poor appetite and intake, nausea, vomiting, inflammation of the mucous membranes in the mouth and dehydration. The extents of the side effects are dependent upon the type of drug used, how it is given, the dosage, and the length of treatment.

Parenteral or Enteral Nutrition for Patients with Advanced Cancer

The use of either parenteral or enteral nutrition in patients with advanced cancer which has been deemed incurable remains a point of debate. The patient and their family's desires for specialized nutrition support along with the risks and benefits of therapy and prognosis should be weighed carefully prior to initiation of therapy. Some patients with advanced cancer such as inoperable tumors of the bowel may actually have improved quality of life with specialized nutrition support. Patients who are not expected to survive more than 3 months are not usually candidates for enteral or parenteral nutrition. Each case is different and should be evaluated appropriately.

Dietary Supplements

According to the Dietary Supplement Health and Education act (DSHEA), a dietary supplement is any product used as part of the diet which contains a vitamin, mineral, herb or amino acid. Dietary supplements also include any metabolite, constituent or extract of any the items previously named. The Food and Drug Administration (FDA) is responsible for making sure that products sold as dietary supplements do not cause significant harm to the consumer if taken as recommended on the label. The manufactures of the products do not need to provide any safety data of their own. Extreme care must be taken when considering such products due to ineffective regulation.

Dietary Supplements Recommendations

Pregnant or lactating women should not take dietary supplements unless recommended by their physician due to potential and unknown side effects to the baby. Infants, children, chronically ill and the elderly should also avoid dietary supplements. Encourage patients to report all supplement use to their physician. If the patient chooses to take supplements, select products that are known to be safe and of high quality, and to follow label directions carefully for dosing instructions. Patients should be educated on using caution when interpreting information obtained from the Internet and in health food stores. Patients should be monitored for any adverse events resulting from the use of dietary supplements including side effects and interaction with prescribed medications or laboratory tests. Patients need to be reminded that products labeled as natural are not necessarily safe.

Use of Breast Milk in Premature Infants

Breast milk is the ideal food for premature infant nutrition. Breast milk is easily digested, the protein is easily absorbed, and the renal solute load is low. Breast milk contains antibodies and immune factors important to the premature baby's development. Breast milk may also be protective against necrotizing enterocolitis. There are many benefits to the mom as well including bonding and a chance to feel like she is contributing to her baby's care. Breast milk, however, does not provide complete nutrition for preterm infants. Human milk fortifiers need to be added to increase calories, protein, calcium, phosphorus, and vitamin D along with many other vitamins and minerals required to meet the increased needs for growth.

Infant Formulas

- Cow's milk based formulas can be used for most term babies with a normally functioning GI tract
- Soy based formulas can be used for vegetarians or who have a documented allergy to cow's milk. It should be noted that many babies with an allergy to cow's milk protein are also allergic to soy therefore caution must be used when initiating soy formula. Soy formula can also be used with lactose deficiency and is indicated for galactosemia.

- Protein hydrolysate formulas can be used for babies with a sensitivity to intact protein or for malabsorption
- Free amino acid based formulas such as Neocate or Elecare for severe protein allergy

Premature Infant Formula

A premature infant formula is indicated for infants with gestational age less than 34 weeks and/or weight less than 2 kilograms. This type of infant formula is specially designed to meet the elevated needs these infants have for rapid growth. This formula contains higher amounts calories and protein. Extra calcium, phosphorus and vitamin D are added for bone development. Zinc and other vitamins are added to help with growth and to prevent deficiency due to reduced stores of many of the vitamins and minerals. The fat source in premature formulas is mainly MCT for improved absorption due to lower levels of pancreatic enzymes. The carbohydrate source is glucose and lactose.

Terms Describing Enteral Formulas

The definitions are as follows:

- Polymeric- a general term used for an enteral formula containing intact protein, complex carbohydrates and long chain fats. This type of formula is used for patients with a normally functioning GI tract.
- Disease specific- formulas designed for the impairment of lung, kidney, liver, glucose control or for patients with trauma or reduced immune functions. These products can be expensive and research has not conclusively shown benefits for all specialized products.
- Modular- single nutrient additives such an intact protein powder, carbohydrate in the form of glucose polymers or fat such as vegetable oil or MCT oil that are added to formulas to change the nutrient composition.
- Chemically defined or hydrolyzed- these formulas are also called semi-elemental. These formulas are peptide-based, lower in fat, lactose free and contain a partially hydrolyzed carbohydrate source. These formulas are used for patients with impairment of the GI tract to help aid in digestion and absorption. There is a higher cost associated with this type of product.
- Elemental- formulas that contain 100% free amino acids, are very low in fat and contain minimal reside. The osmolality of these products is high and may affect tolerance. These formulas are indicated for patients with severe GI compromise. These formulas are costly to use and should only be used if medically necessary

Chemically Defined or Semi Elemental and Elemental Products

Examples of products are as follows and note that the list is not all inclusive:

- Chemically defined/Semi Elemental Formulas- Impact Glutamine (Novartis), Peptinex (Novartis), Vital HN and Optimental (Ross), Peptamen (Nestle),
- Elemental Formulas- Vivonex Plus (Novartis), f.a.a (Nestle)

- Formulas for Liver Disease- Hepatic Aid II (B. Braun), NutriHep (Nestle)
- Formulas for Glucose Intolerance- Glucerna Select (Ross), Diabetisource AC (Novartis), Nutren Glytrol (Nestle)
- Immune Enhanced Formulas-Impact (Novartis), Crucial (Nestle)
- Modular Products-ProPass (Hormel Health), ProCel (Global Unlimited), Resource Beneprotein (Novartis), Karo syrup, MCT Oil, Corn oil, Microlipid (Novartis), Resource Benefiber (Novartis)

Enteral Products

Examples of products are as follows and note that the list is not all inclusive:

- Standard polymeric- Isocal (Novartis), Osmolite (Ross), Nutren (Nestle)
- Fiber containing- Jevity (Ross), Ultracal (Novartis), Nutren 1.0 with Fiber (Nestle)
- Calorically Dense- Boost Plus (Mead Johnson), Ensure Plus HN (Ross), Nutren 1.5 (Nestle), Deliver 2.0 (Mead Johnson), Twocal HN (Ross)
- High Protein Formulas- Replete (Nestle), Promote or Promote with Fiber (Ross), Ultracal (Mead Johnson)
- Renal Formulas- Nepro or Suplena (Ross), Nutren Renal (Nestle), Novasource Renal (Novartis)
- Pulmonary Formulas- Novasource Pulmonary (Novartis), Oxepa and Pulmocare (Ross), Nutren Pulmonary (Nestle)

Water Content of Enteral Formulas and Osmolality

Water is a large component of enteral formulas. Standard, isotonic formulas usually contain 80-85% water while calorically dense formulas contain approximately 70% water. Additional water needs to be provided to most patients receiving enteral nutrition to ensure adequate hydration. Osmolality is the concentration of a solution. It is measured as milliosmoles per kilogram of water (mOsm/kg). Isotonic formulas have an osmolality of approximately 300 mOsm/kg whereas calorically dense formulas can range from 500-700 mOsm/kg. The more hydrolyzed to elemental the formula is, the greater the osmolality will be. For example, a free amino acid based formula will have an osmolality of approximately 600 mOsm/kg whereas an intact protein formula will have an osmolality of approximately 300 mOsm/kg.

Sources of Macronutrients in Polymeric Formulas and Chemically Defined/Hydrolyzed Formulas

The carbohydrate source for polymeric formulas can include corn syrup solids, hydrolyzed cornstarch, sucrose, fructose or maltodextrin. For chemically defined formulas, the carbohydrate source is typically cornstarch, hydrolyzed cornstarch, maltodextrin or fructose. The protein source for polymeric formulas may include casein, sodium caseinate, whey protein concentrate, milk protein concentrate, or soy protein concentrate. For chemically defined formulas, the protein source may include hydrolyzed whey protein, hydrolyzed casein, crystalline L-amino acids, or soy protein isolate. Fat sources for polymeric formulas can vary widely but the most commonly used sources are soybean, corn, canola and high oleic sunflower oil. For chemically defined formulas, the fat source is generally MCT, soybean, safflower or soy lecithin.

Formula Designed for Use with Patients with Diabetes or Glucose Intolerance

Enteral formulas that were designed specifically for blood glucose management contain approximately 30-40% of the calories from carbohydrate and contain various types of fiber. These formulas typically contain 40-50% of the calories as fat. The American Diabetes Association recommends that carbohydrates provide approximately 45-65% of total calories and approximately 30% of total calories as fat. The nutrient composition of these formulas is not parallel with the recommendations. The higher fat content of these products may delay gastric emptying which may already be an issue for patients with gastroparesis as complication of diabetes. The American Diabetes Association recommends using a standard formula containing 50% of the calories as carbohydrate or a lower carbohydrate formula if indicated. It may be prudent to begin with a standard formula and monitor blood glucose levels closely adding insulin when necessary to achieve glycemic control. A lower carbohydrate formula could be used as the next step if glucose levels cannot be controlled otherwise.

Sources of Fiber Commonly Used in Fiber Containing Formulas

Fiber is added to many enteral formulas. It is digested by the bacteria in the colon to produce short chain fatty acids, which are important to intestinal health. The fiber source is typically a blend of soluble and insoluble fiber. Most products contain a type of soy fiber. Some formulas contain fructooligosaccharides (FOS), which promote large bowel health and help to increase the amount of good bacteria in the colon. Soluble fiber may help top reduce diarrhea while insoluble fiber increases the bulk of the stool and slows transit time in the intestines. Patients who are critically ill and are receiving medications that may slow GI function should be closely monitored for tolerance to fiber containing formulas.

Immune Enhanced Formulas

Immune enhanced enteral formulas contain added glutamine, nucleotides, arginine, eicosapentanoic acid, docosahexanoic acid and arachidonic acid. All of these substrates have been shown to have a possible role in the immune process. The theory behind the addition of these substrates is that infection rates will be reduced and the immune response will be improved. Other possible benefits may include the positive effect on wound healing, improvement in gut function and modifying the stress response. The use of immune enhanced enteral formulas is not without controversy. Studies have varied widely in their designs making it difficult to compare results. Further research is needed that include well designed clinical trials studying a large population using the same combination of immune enhancing substrates. Information on dosing, combination of substrates, duration of therapy, and type of patient who will receive the largest benefit still needs to be definitively determined.

Formulas Designed for Patients with Liver Failure

Formulas designed for patients with liver disease contain higher amounts of branched chain amino acids (BCAA) and lower amounts of aromatic amino acids (AAA). The theory behind this is that in liver failure, the body is less able to deaminate amino acids and metabolic disarray can occur. AAA builds up in the blood while BCAA are reduced. AAA are thought to cross the blood- brain barrier and cause additional changes in mental status. Research has not effectively shown a benefit to BCAA enriched formulas compared to traditional therapy using lactulose or neomycin. Other studies have shown a benefit to BCAA enriched formulas in patients with advanced cirrhosis. Additional research needs to be conducted but, in the meantime, routine use of BCAA enriched formulas is discouraged because of the high cost involved as well as well as the fact that long term protein restriction is not recommended for these patients. The product if used, should be done under close medical supervision.

Formulas Appropriate for Renal Patients

Formulas for patients with renal failure contain lower amounts of sodium, potassium and phosphorus for better management of these electrolytes because of impaired excretion in renal failure. The water content of these formulas is also reduced due to volume issues commonly seen with renal failure. The amount of protein provided is dependent upon whether the patient requires a protein restriction. For patients not receiving a form of dialysis or for whom delaying the start of dialysis is warranted, a formula lower in protein is indicated. For patients receiving a form of dialysis, protein requirements can increase to 1.2-2 grams/kg and will require the use of a product with higher amounts of protein. A standard formula may not be appropriate for all patients receiving dialysis due to possible fluid or electrolyte concerns. Modular products are available to help to meet the patients specialized needs.

Enteral Formula Selection for a Patient with Adult Respiratory Distress Syndrome

Patients with Adult Respiratory Distress Syndrome (ARDS) or respiratory failure from some other cause should not be overfed. Providing too many calories may promote carbon dioxide retention and make vent weaning more difficult. There are products available that are lower in carbohydrate and higher in fat designed to reduce carbon dioxide production, however, studies have not conclusively proved this to be beneficial. Additionally, the higher amounts of fat in these types of formulas may delay gastric emptying and cause problems with tolerance. Other studies have shown that excessive calories have a bigger impact on increased carbon dioxide production than carbohydrate intake. In fact, underfeeding using a standard, polymeric formula may be best option for nutrition support during vent weaning. Other studies are looking at the use of omega-3 fatty acids and their effect on ARDS.

Use of Dextrose and Amino Acids as a Macronutrient Source in PN Solutions

Dextrose provides 3.4 kcal/gram. This differs from carbohydrate that provides 4 kcal/gram because dextrose is in its hydrous form as dextrose monohydrate. Dextrose concentrations can range from 2.5% to 70%. Higher dextrose concentrations contribute higher osmolarity and require the use of a central vein for any concentration greater than10%. Crystalline amino acids are used for PN solutions and range in concentration form 3-20%. The most common solutions used are 8.5 and 10% for compounding. Amino acids contribute 4 kcal/gram if used as calories. Amino acid solutions provide a mix of essential and non- essential amino acids.

Benefits of Using an Inline Filter When Infusing PN Solutions

The use of inline filters when infusing TPN solutions is recommended by the Food and Drug Administration and should be part of nursing policy. Various sized filters are available but the general purpose of filter use to help remove particles that may obstruct pulmonary capillaries. Filters are also responsible for trapping microorganisms and air emboli. A size 0.22-micron filter can be used for PN solutions that do not include lipid emulsion as this size filter will trap the fat molecules and clog the filter. A larger size such as 1.2-micron filter can be used for 3- in-1 PN solutions although this size filter is less effective at filtering microorganisms.

Use of Intravenous Fat Emulsions in PN Solutions

IV fat emulsions are a concentrated energy source and also provide essential fatty acids. IVFE are comprised of long chain fatty acids- soy based or a soy-safflower mix. IVFE contain egg yolk and glycerin. IVFE are available as 10%, 20% and 30% emulsions although 30% is used for compounding PN only. Glycerol in the IVFE provides additional calories. 10% emulsion provides 1.1 kcal/ml and 20% provides 2.0 kcal/ml. IVFE have a 12 hour limit for hanging because of the potential for bacterial contamination when infused separately form the dextrose and amino acids. The maximum IVFE infusion rate is 0.11 grams/kg/hour. If this rate is exceeded, side effects may include elevated triglycerides or potential for infection.

Use of Glutamine and Carnitine to PN Solutions

Glutamine is considered to be a conditionally essential amino acid during metabolic stress. It is used as the preferred fuel source of the gut and may help protect gut integrity. Glutamine is unstable in IV solution and is not currently commercially available for use in the United States. It is available for enteral use. Carnitine is involved in the metabolism of long chain fatty acids and the transport of fatty acids into the mitochondria for use as energy. Patients at risk for carnitine deficiency include preterm infants, patients receiving hemodialysis, and patients with liver disease. An IV form of carnitine is available to treat deficiency.

Electrolyte Salts Available for Adding to PN Solutions

Sodium and potassium are available as acetate or phosphate salts. Chloride is available as sodium or potassium chloride. The preferred form of calcium is calcium gluconate and the preferred form of magnesium is magnesium sulfate. These electrolytes are added based on serum electrolyte levels as well as acid base balance.

Products Available for Vitamins and Trace Element Administration

Injectable multivitamins are available for adults and children. This product contains vitamins A, D, E, K, ascorbic acid, thiamin, riboflavin, niacin, pantothentic acid, pyridoxine, vitamin B12, biotin, and folate. Many vitamins are also available for single nutrient injections. Multivitamins should be infused within 24 hours. Vitamin loss can occur due to photodegradation. Trace elements can be given as a concentrate with the dose geared towards adults, children or neonates. Trace element concentrate typically contains forms of zinc, manganese, chromium, copper and selenium. Some facilities also have the trace elements available as single dose injections.

Use of Specialty Amino Acid Solutions Available for Liver Failure

In liver failure, amino acid solutions such as HepatAmine or Hepatasol may be indicated for patients with advanced cirrhosis and hepatic encephalopathy. These formulations contain a mix of essential and non-essential amino acids but contain higher amounts of branched chain amino acids (BCAA) and lower amounts of aromatic amino acids (AAA). The theory is that increased amounts of AAA cross the blood-brain barrier and contribute to altered mental status. This type of formulation is very expensive and its efficacy has not been conclusively documented.

Use of Specialty Amino Acid Solutions in Renal Failure and Metabolic Stress

Specialty amino acid solutions are more costly than standard amino acid solutions and should be used only when clinically indicated. In renal failure, amino acid solutions such as Aminess, RenAmin, and Aminosyn RF provide mainly essential amino acids which cannot be produced in the body. There does not appear to be any major benefit to using a renal formulation and patients may benefit more from the use of a standard amino acid solution in reduced amounts. Specialty amino acid solutions are also available for metabolically stressed patients such as trauma, burns or other hypermetabolic state. Products such as BranchAmine provide increased amounts of branched chain amino acids (BCAA), which are theorized to be helpful during periods of stress because BCAA are the preferred fuel for skeletal muscles. Studies have not supported routine use of this type of product for improving morbidity and mortality.

Total Nutrient Admixture System

Total Nutrient Admixture (TNA) is a system for compounding PN solutions to include dextrose, amino acids, fat emulsion and all electrolyte, vitamins, minerals and trace elements into one solution. This is also referred to as a 3-in-1 solution. The advantage to this system is that there is a reduced risk for bacterial contamination. Once the PN solution is hung and administration begins, there should not be any additional entries into this port for the next 24 hours. TNA system is more cost effective and it is easier for the pharmacy to prepare. There is less nursing time involved with this system. IV fat emulsion may also be better tolerated because of the longer infusion time (24 hours versus 12 hours if the fat emulsion is infused separately).

Specialized Amino Acid Solutions Available for Pediatric Use

Specialized pediatric amino acid formulations are recommended for infants and young children. Adult standard solutions do not meet the needs of an infant and should not be used on an infant less than 1 year of age. These pediatric solutions contain conditionally essential amino acids that are not produced in amounts adequate enough to meet the infant's requirements. These amino acids are tyrosine, taurine, and histidine. Glutamine is also conditionally essential however, an IV form that is stable in solution is not available. The amino acid composition is designed to produce an amino acid profile similar to that of a breast-fed baby. Phenylalanine, methionine, and glycine are reduced to prevent the infant from receiving too much of these amino acids. Examples of pediatric crystalline amino acids solutions are Trophamine and Aminosyn PF. Cysteine must be added at 40 mg/ gram of protein when Trophamine is used.

2-in-1 Formulations for PN Solution

The 2-in-1 PN solution is also known as the traditional formulation. It incorporates all PN components into one solution with the exception of the IV fat emulsion (IVFE). The IVFE is infused separately called a piggyback infusion. The IVFE should not hang for longer than12 hours due to the risk for fungal or bacterial contamination. Patients who receive separate IVFE may experience an increase is serum triglyceride levels because the infusion rate is faster than over a 24 hour period and the body may be less able to clear the lipids from the blood stream. The advantage to this type of system is that it allows for higher concentrations of calcium and phosphorus to be added. It also reduces the chance for medication incompatibilities and with a clear solution, it easier to monitor for precipitation.

Total Nutrient Admixture System

There are disadvantages to the TNA system. One disadvantage is that because of the creamy color of the solution, it is more difficult to monitor for any precipitates that may occur such as with calcium and phosphate. TNA requires the use of a larger inline filter and catheter occlusion is more common. Larger inline filters are not as effective in filtering out bacterial contaminants. The TNA solution is less stable once the IV fat emulsion is added and many medications are not compatible with lipid. The TNA solution can be unstable if the dextrose or amino acids concentrations are too low. This type of system may be more costly for a facility where only a few TNA solutions are prepared daily.

Labeling Procedures for PN Solutions

The label on PN solutions is an important safety feature. Proper labeling can help reduce errors that may occur when a patient transfers from one facility to another but ideally should include communication between pharmacists at both facilities. The best labeling method is for a 24 hour infusion to record the quantity of all components provided for the day. For institutions that compound PN solutions in one-liter bags, the label should list the components per container. This should help to reduce confusion regarding the final concentrations of all components. It should also help to prevent overdosing of electrolytes. Both per day and per container additives can be listed on the same label in clearly marked columns. The weight used for dosing should also be listed on the label along with the route of administration, infusion rate, and duration. It should also include the beyond use dating and the administration date. Any added overfill should be clearly stated.

Safety Measures for Compounded Sterile Products

The safe preparation of a PN solution is of utmost importance. Guidelines have been established defining the "beyond use dating" which is a relatively new term used to replace the term expiration date. The beyond use dating is applied to various types of solutions while at room temperature and under refrigeration. Automated compounding devices are devices used as a tool for ensuring the accuracy of the dosing of components in the PN solution. For PN solutions that are made without the use of an automated compounding device, a different pharmacist should verify the syringes used to prepare the solution for accuracy. Automated compounding devices have built in safety features to verify the correct dose of each component and will compare the actual weight of the final solution with the expected weight calculated by the device. Other procedures should be in place that addresses the proper transport and handling of the PN solution.

Compatibility

The term compatibility typically refers to the physical and chemical interactions between components in PN solutions and whether precipitates will form in solution. Precipitates can be in the form of crystals such as a calcium phosphate precipitate or as a separation of components such as oil and water. Often times the limiting factor for compatibility is the addition of the lipid emulsion, which affects the compatibility of many medications. The addition of iron dextran to TNA is not compatible with lipid and always causes instability. Iron dextran should always be added to a lipid free PN solution.

Stability

The term stability means the quality of a solution being resistant to changes. There are a variety of factors that can cause a solution to become unstable. Multivitamin injections should be added just before administration of the PN solution because it is not stable if added more than 24 hours before use. Photodegradation, which means the breaking down of the solution when exposed to light, primarily affects vitamins including the B vitamins, vitamin A and K. The pH level of the PN solution is very important for stability. A pH level less than 5 or greater than10 may cause the solution to "crack" or separate yielding it unsafe for use. The crystalline amino acid solution exerts the most influence on the final pH of the PN solution. A Maillard reaction describes the process that causes a brown coloration to the solution because of the interaction between carbohydrates, certain amino acids, and temperature.

Calcium and Phosphate Compatibility

Calcium and phosphate compatibility is one of the most serious concerns when compounding a PN solution. If calcium and phosphate are not added in the correct amounts, precipitation can occur and crystals can form. These crystals can potentially enter the pulmonary veins causing pulmonary emboli and possible death. There are many factors that affect the compatibility including the concentration of amino acids, the type of amino acid solution used, the type of calcium salt used, the dextrose concentration, the temperature of the solution, and the pH. PN solutions with lower pH levels are less likely to precipitate. In the neonatal population, l-cysteine is added because it is a semi-essential amino acid and also serves to lower the pH. Higher amounts of calcium and phosphate are needed in this population to help prevent metabolic bone disease. Pharmacists have tools available to assist with evaluating calcium and phosphate solubility including solubility curves, computer software used in conjunction with automated compounding devices and visual assessment of the calcium prescription compared to normal recommendations.

Medications Not Compatible with PN Solutions

When considering whether certain medications are compatible with a PN solution, the use of TNA or a transitional dextrose-amino acid solution needs to be determined. Some medications can be added to the solution while others are given at the Y site. Common medications that are incompatible with both types of solutions include acyclovir, amphotericin, cyclosporine, ganciclovir, and midazolam. The registered pharmacist and the Nutrition Support Team should be actively involved in determining the appropriateness of medications being ordered for use with patients receiving PN therapy. Patients with limited access may need to have the TPN infusion held for the administration of certain medications through the same line.

Calculating the Osmolarity of a PN Solution

A simple method of calculating the osmolarity of a PN solution based on a liter of solution is: osmolarity of dextrose is ~5 mOsm/gram, amino acids is ~10 mOsm/gram, and electrolytes contribute 1 mOsm per mEq. Lipids are isotonic and contribute minimally to the final osmolarity. An alternate calculation uses the same dextrose and amino acid calculations but takes twice the sum of the calcium, magnesium, sodium and potassium per liter to calculate the osmolarity. A reminder that these equations are just estimates and compounding software can more accurately calculate the osmolarity of a solution.

NSC Practice Test

1. Which of the following clinical parameters is LEAST likely to be an indicator of a nutritionally at-risk patient in an acute care hospital?

a. 5% unplanned weight loss in a 1-month period
b. Inadequate nutrition for 10 days
c. Intentional weight loss of 15% over a 6-month period in an obese individual
d. Extensive resection of the colon due to cancer

2. Which of the following anthropometric methods is LEAST useful in nutrition assessment in an ICU setting?

a. Triceps skinfold
b. Body mass index
c. Estimating ideal body weight using height and Hamwi equation
d. Comparing actual weight to either ideal weight or usual weight

3. When performing a nutrition-focused physical examination, the presence of scaly, dry skin may indicate

a. vitamin A toxicity.
b. essential fatty acid deficiency.
c. cholesterol deficiency.
d. protein deficiency.

4. Which of the following medications is LEAST likely to cause weight gain?

a. Paxil
b. Elavil
c. Wellbutrin
d. Prozac

5. When diagnosing malnutrition in an acutely ill patient, the LEAST valid marker to use would be

a. unplanned weight loss of 8% in a 4-month period.
b. body mass index of 16 kg/m2.
c. poor wound healing.
d. serum albumin of 2.5 g/dL.

6. Which of the following is the best tool for assessing a patient with chronic liver disease and ascites?

a. Weight for height
b. Subjective Global Assessment
c. Albumin and prealbumin
d. Nitrogen balance

7. What is the appropriate weight to use for calculations for an obese patient with chronic kidney disease?

a. Dry weight
b. Adjusted dry weight
c. Ideal weight
d. Actual weight

8. A patient is taking the anti-HIV drug Zerit. This drug is likely to cause

a. lipodystrophy
b. AIDS wasting syndrome
c. malnutrition
d. metabolic syndrome

9. Which of the following best describes the timing for initiation of an enteral feeding protocol for a patient with a traumatic brain injury?

a. Within 24 hours
b. Within 48 hours
c. As soon as a nasogastric tube can be placed
d. Once bowel sounds are distinctly heard

10. What is a reasonable level of protein for a patient with a 50% TBSA in the early post-burn period?

a. 1.0-1.2 grams per kg
b. 1.2-1.5 grams per kg
c. 1.5-2.0 grams per kg
d. 2.0-2.5 grams per kg

11. A patient with COPD is currently on mechanical ventilation for respiratory failure with the goal of weaning in the next several days. He is at 85% of his ideal body weight and 95% of his usual body weight. What would be the best weight to use for calculating energy requirements?

a. Ideal weight
b. Usual weight
c. Actual weight
d. Adjusted weight

12. How many kilocalories does 2280 cc of a D15% 4% amino acid and 3% intralipid 3-in-1 TNA solution contain?

a. 2140 kcal
b. 2207 kcal
c. 2345 kcal
d. 2413 kcal

13. A 70-year-old man who has a history of esophageal cancer is doing well nutritionally on gastrostomy tube feedings. He is 5'10" and weighs 160 pounds. His weight has been stable on 2000 kcal per day in the form of 1 kcal/cc formula. He has also been receiving an additional 500 mL of water per day. He is changing his tube feeding regimen from a 1 kcal/cc formulation to a 1.25-kcal formulation in order to provide more free time from the G tube feedings. His caloric intake should remain the same. How much water will he need to receive in addition to the formula after the change to maintain the same level of hydration? (Assume 1.0 kcal/cc formulation is 84% water and 1.25 kcal/cc formulation is 80% water)

a. 700 mL
b. 840 mL
c. 900 mL
d. 1280 mL

14. A patient admitted with a history of chronic alcohol abuse and possible Wernicke encephalopathy will require immediate supplementation with

a. thiamine.
b. potassium.
c. phosphate.
d. magnesium.

15. What is the preferred method of initial nutrition support for a patient admitted with severe pancreatitis?

a. Nasogastric tube with standard formula
b. Nasojejunal tube with a standard formula
c. Parenteral nutrition
d. NPO until pain subsides, then allow diet to advance

16. Which of the following statements is most correct regarding medical nutrition therapy for patients with high output enterocutaneous fistulas?

a. Patients with a mid-jejunal fistula can easily be fed with enteral nutrition using a PEG/J tube.
b. Parenteral nutrition is always required for enterocutaneous fistulas.
c. Patients with distal ileum or colonic fistulas cannot be fed enterally until the fistula is closed.
d. Patients with a proximal fistula can be fed using enteral nutrition if the nasojejunal tube is placed beyond the site of the fistula.

17. A patient with gastroparesis has been receiving appropriate medical nutrition therapy for an oral diet as well as prokinetic medication. Her nutritional status is not improving, as evidenced by failure to gain weight and continued nausea and vomiting. What is the next step for feeding this patient?

a. Use a surgically placed gastrostomy tube with initiation of elemental formula.
b. Allow the patient to continue an oral diet while a nasojejunal tube is placed and a polymeric formula is started nocturnally.
c. Make the patient strict NPO and begin enteral nutrition using a polymeric formula through a nasojejunal tube.
d. Begin parenteral nutrition immediately.

18. A patient has a clogged NG tube. Flushing gently with warm water has not resolved the obstruction. What would be the most effective next step to take to try to clear the obstruction?

a. Aggressive flushing with cranberry juice
b. A mixture of pancreatic enzymes and water or sodium bicarbonate flushed through the tube
c. Gentle flushing with a cola product
d. Passing a thin stiff wire through the tube to try to break up the clot

19. Which of the following antibiotics would most likely require an alternation in feeding schedule for a patient with a J tube?

a. Ciprofloxacin
b. Amoxicillin
c. Cefazolin
d. Azithromycin

20. A patient experienced radical neck dissection 1 week ago due to cancer. He had a gastrostomy tube placed during surgery and had been receiving a standard polymeric formulation. He is now diagnosed with a chyle leak based on a triglyceride level of 160 mg/dL of the pleural fluid. A chest tube is placed for drainage and initial treatment will be conservative to determine if the leak will close spontaneously. The first 2 days of drainage yield over 750 mL per day. Which of the following is the most appropriate nutritional recommendation?

a. Recommend that tube feedings be held for a few days to determine if drainage will be reduced.
b. Recommend total parenteral nutrition.
c. Continue the same gastrostomy feedings that he was receiving prior to diagnosis of chyle leak.
d. Recommend that the formula be changed to a low-fat semi-elemental formula.

21. The following patients have all had extensive bowel resections requiring long-term TPN. In which patient is it most appropriate to recommend a change to a cyclic TPN schedule?

a. A 15-year-old girl with a history of hypoglycemia
b. A 30-year-old woman stable on mechanical ventilation
c. A 6-month-old stable infant getting ready for discharge
d. A 73-year-old man with a history of CHF receiving intensive physical and occupational therapy

22. A 60-year-old man is admitted with dysphagia and a 15-pound weight loss. He is diagnosed with esophageal cancer. Before treatment is to begin, he has a portacath and a PEJ tube placed in preparation for chemotherapy and radiation prior to surgery. He has good bowel sounds and is having bowel movements. He is not able to eat more than sips of liquids throughout the day. The dietitian has estimated his calorie needs to be approximately 2275 kcals (35 kcal/kg), 98 grams protein (1.5 grams/kg), and 1950 cc fluid (30 cc/kg). Which of the following is the most appropriate plan for initiating and advancing tube feedings?

a. Start 20 cc/hour of elemental formula and advance by 20 cc/hour every 4 to 6 hours as tolerated until goal rate of 95 cc/hour is reached.
b. Start bolus feedings of standard isotonic fiber containing formula, 120 cc, every 4 hours for 24 hours. On the second day increase the bolus feedings to 240 cc per feeding every 4 hours. On the third day increase to goal of 360 cc every 4 hours.
c. Start 30 cc/hour of a standard isotonic formula and advance by 30 cc/hour per day until goal of 90 cc/hour is reached.
d. Start 25 cc/hour of standard isotonic fiber containing formula and advance by 25 cc/hour every 6 to 8 hours, as tolerated, until the goal of 90 cc/hour is reached.

23. A 38-year-old woman is transferred to the general surgery floor from an outside hospital with a small bowel obstruction. She has been receiving a 2-in-1 central TPN solution consisting of 1970 kcal (390 grams dextrose, 70 grams protein in 1550 ml) with 250 ml 20% lipids. Her current weight is 59 kg and her height is 5'6". Laboratory data is remarkable for blood glucose of 250 mg/dL. Upon reassessment, which of the following is the most appropriate step to take?

a. Reduce dextrose concentration.
b. Reduce total calories.
c. Reduce both total calories and dextrose concentration.
d. Reduce dextrose concentration and increase lipids.

24. A patient had a lung transplant 1 week ago. She was moderately malnourished prior to transplant. She has been receiving a high-protein polymeric tube feeding via a nasogastric tube at goal rate with good tolerance. She is beginning an oral diet. What is the next step in treatment?

a. Discontinue tube feedings when oral diet meets at least 50% of her nutritional needs.
b. Change to nocturnal tube feedings when she is consuming at least 50% of her nutritional needs.
c. Continue 24-hour tube feedings until she is consuming 80% of her nutritional needs.
d. Hold tube feedings for 3 days to see if she is able to meet her nutritional needs with an oral diet.

25. When making decisions about artificial nutrition and hydration (ANH) for a patient with advanced dementia, which of the following takes precedence?

a. Whatever the patient decides
b. The surrogate decision maker
c. Health care proxy
d. Advance directive, such as living will

26. What is the estimated water deficit for 70-year-old man with a weight of 80 kg and a serum sodium level of 156 mEq/L?

a. 1 liter
b. 3 liters
c. 5 liters
d. 7 liters

27. Which of the following is the LEAST likely cause of diarrhea in a hospitalized patient receiving enteral nutrition?

a. Soluble fiber
b. *C. difficile*
c. Elixir form of medications
d. Magnesium containing medications

28. A patient receiving central TPN and IV Diprivan should be closely monitored for

a. hyperglycemia.
b. hypercapnia.
c. hypertriglyceridemia.
d. hypercholesterolemia.

29. Which of the following is NOT indicative of the metabolic response to refeeding syndrome?

a. Insulin secretion causing an increase in glucose uptake in the cells leading to alterations in glucose metabolism
b. Sodium and fluid retention secondary to SIADH
c. An intracellular shift of phosphorus into the cells causing a reduction in oxygen release to cells, thus impairing respiratory function
d. Cardiac alterations such as EKG changes or arrhythmias due to hypokalemia

30. Metabolic alkalosis may be caused by

a. renal failure.
b. fasting.
c. diarrhea.
d. severe vomiting.

31. Respiratory acidosis is most always caused by

a. over-aggressive diuretic therapy.
b. a decrease in alveolar ventilation.
c. renal failure.
d. ingestion of toxins that lead to lactic acidosis.

32. Which of the following is the LEAST likely cause of PN associated liver disease (PNALD) in adults?

a. Overfeeding of total calories from TPN
b. Excessive dextrose administration
c. Excessive lipid administration
d. Excessive amino acid administration

33. In a patient with significant risk factors for aspiration, which of the following is the initial step to reduce the risk?

a. Add blue food coloring to the enteral feeding formula.
b. Monitor residuals and hold tube feeding for residuals greater than 100 mL.
c. Elevate the head of the bed 45 degrees.
d. Change to an elemental or semi-elemental formulation.

34. A 35-year-old woman has been on home total nutrient admixture (TNA) regimen for 4 months for gastrointestinal issues related to Crohn disease. She is not able to take any food enterally due to diarrhea. She has just been diagnosed with iron deficiency anemia. Which recommendation is most appropriate for repletion?

a. Give IV iron dextran after a test dose to establish that she is safe to receive it.
b. Add iron dextran to the total nutrient admixture.
c. Add sodium ferric gluconate to total nutrient admixture.
d. Begin an oral iron regimen taken at the same time as vitamin C to enhance absorption.

35. Which of the following is NOT a symptom of catheter-related thrombosis?

a. Ability to infuse into the line but not aspirate blood out of it
b. Frequent pump alarms
c. Swelling of the facial area, including around the eyes
d. Rapid heart rate and shortness of breath

36. A patient is receiving enteral nutrition through an NG tube and is experiencing nausea, vomiting, abdominal pain, and a feeling of choking. This may be a symptom of

a. formula intolerance.
b. anxiety surrounding presence of NG tube.
c. tube displacement.
d. post-nasal drip.

37. What would be an INAPPROPRIATE plan for initiation of nutrition support in patient at risk for the refeeding syndrome?

a. Recommend BEE plus 20%.
b. Recommend 50% of calculated energy requirements using the Harris Benedict equation plus a factor of 1.3-1.5.
c. Recommend 20 kcal/kg.
d. Any of the above would be an appropriate starting point.

38. To help prevent the development of PN-associated metabolic bone disease, which of the following is NOT recommended?

a. Make sure protein intake is maximized to the upper end of the estimated range.
b. Ensure adequate acetate is added to the PN solution to correct the presence of metabolic acidosis.
c. Maximize calcium intake to 10-15 mEq per day and phosphorus to 20-40 mmol per day.
d. Maximize magnesium intake to 8-20 mEq per day to maintain normal serum levels.

39. A patient who is stable for 6 months on long-term home TPN should have a comprehensive metabolic panel including electrolytes, BUN, creatinine, albumin, calcium, phosphorus, magnesium and liver function tests, and CBC with differential monitored how frequently?

a. Weekly
b. Biweekly
c. Monthly
d. Semiannually

40. A patient with chronic kidney disease (CKD) receiving hemodialysis who has an intact PTH of 430 pg/mL should receive what form of vitamin D?

a. Ergocalciferol
b. 1,25 -dihydroxyvitamin D
c. 25 -hydroxyvitamin D
d. Cholecalciferol

41. A patient is receiving enteral feedings of a polymeric formula 75 mL/hour through a PEG. Omeprazole is being started in capsule form for GERD. What is the most appropriate way to administer this medication?

a. Open the capsule and dissolve in apple juice. Administer through the PEG, flush with apple juice, then hold tube feedings for 1 hour.
b. Hold tube feedings for 1 hour, open capsule and dissolve in water then administer through the PEG. Flush with additional water, then hold the feeding for another hour.
c. Crush the capsule and dissolve in 30 mL of water and administer through the PEG, followed by water flush.
d. If the patient is able to swallow the capsule, this should be done; otherwise, ask the physician to change to the IV form of the medication.

42. A patient on long-term TPN with total bilirubin levels greater than 3.5 is at potential risk for toxicity of

a. zinc and selenium.
b. selenium and manganese.
c. copper and chromium.
d. manganese and copper.

43. In writing a nutrition support protocol related to peripheral parenteral nutrition (PPN), which of the following statements is NOT supported by evidence-based practice?

a. To reduce the risk for phlebitis, the peripheral cannula should be rotated approximately every 72 hours to a new location.
b. Solutions with an osmolarity between 900-1200 mOsm/L may be safely infused through a midline catheter.
c. PPN should only be selected for patients who require therapy for less than 2 weeks.
d. PPN solutions will generally require a lower dextrose concentration of 5-10% and a final amino acid concentration of 3%.

44. According to the Centers for Disease Control Guidelines for the Prevention of Intravascular Catheter-Related Infections, which of the following is NOT considered an appropriate antiseptic for use in preparing the skin for a catheter site dressing change?

a. Neosporin ointment
b. 70% alcohol
c. Chlorhexidine
d. Tincture of iodine

45. Which is the LEAST preferred site for inserting a central venous catheter (CVC)?

a. Basilic
b. Cephalic
c. Internal jugular
d. Femoral

46. Which of the following is NOT an accurate description of the Patient Self-Determination Act?

a. Legal requirement for health care institutions to provide information to all patients regarding rights surrounding health care decision making
b. Legal requirement that a patient be asked if there is an advance directive and for the documentation in the medical record if there is an advance directive
c. Legal requirement for all patients to have an advance directive upon admission to hospital or nursing home
d. Legal requirement to provide education and training to all staff regarding advance directives

47. Which of the following is NOT a position of The American Society for Enteral and Parenteral Nutrition (A.S.P.E.N.) regarding artificial nutrition and hydration (ANH)?

a. Withholding or withdrawing ANH is never acceptable in the cases of infants or children unless death is imminent within hours.
b. Decisions regarding ANH should be a decision made using a combination of clinical judgment and evidence-based medicine along with input from the patient or family.
c. The perspective of ethnicity, religion, and culture should be taken into account when making decisions regarding ANH.
d. There is most likely a lack of benefit from providing ANH to patients with severe dementia and may contribute some degree of risk to the patient if provided.

48. Which of the following is the LEAST appropriate source to use when applying evidence-based practice (EBP)?

a. Controlled trial without randomization
b. Meta-analysis
c. Cohort study
d. Case-control analysis studied

49. A patient is admitted to the medical ICU with dehydration, decompensated liver disease, end-stage cirrhosis, and acute encephalopathy. He is nonadherent with his lactulose medication at times. The patient is to begin nasogastric tube feedings. The physician is requesting a branched-chain amino-acid based product. Based on evidence-based practice, which of the following is the best step to take?

a. Agree to this recommendation.
b. Provide an alternative recommendation for a polymeric formula that will provide 0.5 grams per kg of protein.
c. Explain to the physician that there have been no studies to document clinical support for this product and it is best used with intractable encephalopathy in patients who are not responsive to aggressive medical management first.
d. Recommend that TPN be initiated.

50. A patient is receiving central TPN with insulin added. She has also been receiving an insulin drip. Blood glucose levels have been stable and an order is written to discontinue the insulin drip. This order does not get implemented immediately, and upon recheck of the patient's glucose level, severe hypoglycemia is discovered with a serum glucose level of 20 mg/dL. This is an example of

a. medication error.
b. adverse occurrence.
c. risk management.
d. sentinel event.

Answer Key and Explanations

1. C: The Joint Commission (formerly the Joint Commission on Accreditation of Healthcare Organizations or JCAHO) mandates that nutrition screening be completed within 24 hours of admission. Risk factors are identified to determine the level of nutritional risk for each patient. Weight is frequently used as a risk factor. An unplanned weight change of more than 10% over a 6-month period or a 5% unplanned change over a 1-month period would be considered a nutritional risk factor. An obese patient who has intentionally lost 15% of his or her body weight would not necessarily be at nutritional risk, especially if patient was following a nutritionally adequate diet. Other risk factors would include a period longer than 7 days of inadequate nutrition; changes in GI function such as nausea, vomiting, or bowel issues; or extensive GI surgery. Many long-term diseases would also affect nutritional status. The use of certain medications, changes in the ability to chew or swallow, and social factors would also influence nutritional status.

2. A: Assessment of body composition using triceps skinfold (TSF) as a measure of subcutaneous fat, and midarm circumference (MAC) and midarm muscle circumference (MAMC) as a measure of lean body mass is not as useful in an ICU setting. One reason for this is because the patient's arm may not be easily accessible in an intensive care setting. A second reason is because the standards for TSF, MAC, and MAMC were developed using healthy individuals who were not hospitalized. Changes in the hydration status of the patient as well as differences in techniques can vary between those who are measuring. Body mass index (BMI) is useful in helping to classify a patient's nutritional status. BMI also has limitations, such as misclassifying patients who have a large amount of muscle as obese. Comparing a patient's current weight to usual weight is fairly useful, especially when coupled with evaluating the reasons for weight loss. Using height and the Hamwi equation can also be useful for comparing the patient to the normal population.

3. B: In a nutrition-focused physical examination, the skin can be very informative to the overall nutritional status of the patient. Dry, scaly skin or dermatitis may be indicative of an essential fatty acid deficiency. Poor wound healing may be indicative of a deficiency of vitamin C, zinc, or protein. The turgor of the skin (ability of the skin to change shape and return to normal) can be a good indicator of hydration status. A pale skin color may be indicative of a deficiency of iron, vitamin B_{12}, or folate. Individuals with high cholesterol levels will sometimes exhibit tiny lumps on the eye lids or elbows. Excessive bruising as seen with the presence of petechiae or ecchymosis may be due to a deficiency of vitamins C or K.

4. C: Most antidepressant medications may cause weight gain and it is important to identify any medications a patient may be taking for depression. The mechanism for this may be multifaceted. There may be a metabolic effect, such as a decrease in metabolic rate. There may also be an increase in appetite related to a medication, causing an increase in caloric intake. It may also be a result of an overall improvement in well-being as a result of depression improving and food intake increasing. Antidepressants such as Wellbutrin, Effexor, and Serzone are least likely to cause an increase in weight. Selective serotonin reuptake inhibitors (SSRI) drugs are more likely to cause weight gain. These include Paxil, Lexapro, Prozac, and Zoloft. MAO inhibitors such as Nardil and Parnate, and tricyclics such as Elavil are also more likely to cause weight gain.

5. D: Revisions are underway for the criteria used to diagnose malnutrition using ICD-10 codes. The use of albumin and pre-albumin as a marker for protein status are typically an unreliable measure. This is due to the fact that in acute illness, albumin and pre-albumin function as inflammatory biomarkers. Inflammation does have negative consequences for nutritional status; however, these markers will not accurately measure visceral protein status. Better indicators of protein status include improvement in weight, strength, and wound healing. Other markers of overall nutrition status are the degree of weight change over a designated period of time and loss of subcutaneous fat or muscle. Compromised nutrient intake would also be a better marker, as would changes in physical function such as hand grip strength.

6. B: Nutrition assessment of a patient with advanced chronic liver disease and ascites is difficult because many of the usual parameters are not reliable. Anthropometric parameters such as weight for height, BMI, and triceps skinfold measurements are affected by fluid status and do not accurately reflect muscle mass or actual weight. Plasma protein status, such as serum albumin or prealbumin, are not useful because they are produced by the liver and do not reflect protein status in liver disease, even in a well-nourished patient. Nitrogen balance studies may not be accurate due to retention of protein in the form of ammonias, as well as the potential for hepatorenal complications affecting nitrogen excretion. The best tool may be subjective global assessment (SGA). This type of tool incorporates a functional and physical examination. Areas that can be evaluated include previous intake, weight history, visible loss of muscle mass, and ability to perform activities of daily living. The presence of other chronic diseases as well as GI symptoms can also be evaluated.

7. B: Anthropometric assessment is an important piece in patients with chronic kidney disease. Many calculations are based on weight, including calorie and protein requirements, medications, and other treatments. Current weight and a history of weight changes are important to document. For non-obese patients, the dry weight should be used for calculations because it reflects metabolically active lean body weight. If a patient is obese or overweight, an adjusted dry body weight should be calculated. According to the National Kidney Foundation KDOQI guidelines, the adjusted dry weight can be calculated using the following equation: adjusted dry weight = dry weight + [(standard body weight - dry weight) x 0.25] where the standard body weight can be obtained using data from NHANES II. Using the adjusted dry body weight will assist with fine tuning energy and protein requirements based on the dry lean body mass to prevent overfeeding.

8. A: Zerit (stavudine) is an anti-HIV drug that is likely to cause lipodystrophy. Protease inhibitors have also been known to cause lipodystrophy. Lipodystrophy is a change in the way the body produces, stores, and utilizes fat. Lipodystrophy can cause fat accumulation in certain areas of the body such as the back of the neck, the abdomen, and breasts in both men and women. This is measured by calculating the waist-to-hip ratio, as well as skin fold measurements and measurements of other areas affected. Lipodystrophy can also cause fat wasting in areas of the body such as the face (causing sunken cheeks and temporal wasting) and loss of fat in the extremities and buttocks. Lipodystrophy can also cause other metabolic abnormalities such as hyperlipidemia, hyperglycemia, and lactic acidosis. Older Caucasian men are more likely to develop lipodystrophy. Individuals who are obese and those that have had HIV for a period of time are also at higher risk for developing this disorder.

9. A: Enteral feeding is always the preferred route of feeding for critically ill patients. With a traumatic brain injury (TBI), feeding intolerance and gastrointestinal reflux are often present. Nasogastric tubes are typically placed without difficulty; however, these are not recommended for early feeding due to the risk of aspiration pneumonia and the likelihood of feeding intolerance. Some patients can tolerate the placement of a nasoenteric tube into the duodenum or jejunum. Early enteral feeding has been shown to be beneficial in the treatment of TBI and should ideally be initiated within the first 24 hours. At least half of the patient's energy and protein requirements should be provided. The theory behind the early initiation of enteral feedings is that it helps to reduce the patient's inflammatory response, which typically peaks around the second week. Early feeding has also been shown to reduce mortality. Early feeding helps to reduce bacterial translocation and stimulates blood flow to the gut.

10. D: There are many equations to predict the amount of protein required for patients with burn injury. A major burn will increase the catabolic rate in the body. In the initial post-burn injury period, approximately 2.0-2.5 grams per kg are required, or approximately 2-25% of total calories. As the burn begins to heal additional protein may be required, especially with large total surface area burns. The provision of high amounts of protein will not prevent catabolism but will assist with achieving anabolism and begin to promote healing. Patient tolerance to an increased protein load should be monitored, watching for azotemia and level of wound healing. Nitrogen balance can be evaluated using the equation: grams of nitrogen – grams of urinary urea nitrogen + 4. Normal renal function and accurate intake and output records are required. An anabolic range of +5 to +10 is the goal during the acute recovery phase.

11. C: Indirect calorimetry is the best way to calculate energy requirements for a patient with respiratory failure and COPD. Many times, this is not an option and the registered dietitian must calculate estimated energy requirements. The provision of too many calories may result in overfeeding, making it more difficult to wean from the ventilator. Overfeeding may be seen with an increase in carbon dioxide production. Underfeeding is not optimal either because it causes catabolism and overall deconditioning in an already compromised patient. For patients who are underweight, actual body weight should be used for calculating energy needs—especially during the weaning process. Ideal body weight should be used for calculations in patients who are at or up to 24% above their ideal body weight. For patients who are 25% or more above ideal body weight, an adjusted body weight should be used. The equation for calculating adjusted ideal body weight is: (actual body weight – ideal body weight) x 0.25 + ideal body weight.

12. B: Many institutions are using a 3-in-1 parenteral nutrition solution, also known as TNA or total nutrient admixtures. In this type of solution, the intravenous fat emulsion is added into the solution instead of being piggybacked into the IV line. TNA incorporates dextrose, amino acids, lipids, electrolytes, vitamins, minerals, and other additives. In this example, the total volume was 2280 cc. Using a 15% dextrose solution, this would provide 342 grams of dextrose. Since dextrose provides 3.4 kcal per gram, the caloric contribution from dextrose is 1163 kcal. Amino acids consisted of 4% of the solution or 91 grams of protein (364 kcal). Lipids at 3% of the solution provide approximately 68 grams of fat. Lipids contain glycerol; therefore, the caloric content is 10 kcal per gram instead of 9 kcal per gram since glycerol contributes a small amount of calories. The caloric content of the lipids is 680 kcal. Total caloric content of the TNA is approximately 2207 kcal.

13. C: The patient is currently receiving 2000 mL × 84% or 1680 mL + 500 mL extra, for a total of 2180 mL of water per day. That same amount should be maintained after the change. The new formula will not be 2000 mL since it is more nutrient dense, so calculate the amount of new formula needed to maintain the same caloric intake: 2000 kcal × 1 mL/1.25 kcal = 1600 mL of the new formula. The new formula is also a different percentage water, so calculate the volume of water contained in a day of the new formula: 1600 mL × 80% = 1280 mL of water. Subtract this from the total water intake to find the amount of additional water needed: 2180 mL – 1280 mL = 900 mL additional water.

14. A: Chronic alcohol abuse can lead to a deficiency of many nutrients. Wernicke encephalopathy can occur as a result of alcohol abuse, inadequate thiamine intake, and impaired thiamine absorption. Signs of a thiamine deficiency include loss of memory, reduced appetite, nausea and vomiting, difficulty sleeping, weakness, and anxiety. As the deficiency progresses, it can lead to confusion, disorientation, hallucinations, and coma. Beriberi is a form of thiamine deficiency with neurological symptoms and cardiac failure. If Wernicke encephalopathy is suspected, immediate treatment with IV thiamine should begin with a gradual shift to oral thiamine after 1-2 weeks. Magnesium typically needs to be supplemented as well because magnesium is a cofactor in many thiamine pathways. Many other nutrients may be deficient as well, including folate, fat-soluble vitamins, zinc, selenium, potassium, and phosphate.

15. B: Acute pancreatitis is caused by chronic alcohol abuse in over 75% of cases. Other reasons for acute pancreatitis include diseases or disorders of the biliary tract, medications, and trauma. A systemic immuno-inflammatory response (SIR) occurs once pancreatitis begins that is consistent with intense pain and cytokine production. Patients become hypermetabolic with skeletal muscle catabolism causing a rapid decline in nutritional status. Research has demonstrated that early enteral nutrition can help with gut integrity and blood flow to the gut, causing secretion of secretory IgA and bile salts to help protect the gut from injury. A nasojejunal tube placed below the ligament of Treitz is the preferred route for enteral feeding. In this case, a standard formula can be initiated. If the patient does not tolerate this type of formula, an elemental or semi-elemental low-fat formula can be tried. Parenteral nutrition is a last resort. An oral diet cannot be started until pain subsides, which often occurs 5-7 days after diagnosis.

16. D: An enterocutaneous (EC) fistula is an opening between 2 surfaces, such as the small and large bowel or the large bowel and skin. EC fistulas can occur as a complication of GI surgery, related to cancer therapy, infection, or abdominal trauma. Managing the medical nutrition of a patient with a fistula is extremely challenging. The route of nutrition for a patient with a fistula is dependent upon the location of the fistula. In most cases, if enteral nutrition is selected as the route, the feeding tube must be placed beyond the location of the fistula to increase the success of feeding. A fistula located in the mid-jejunum may not have success with enteral nutrition. The reason for this is that there may not be enough surface area available for sufficient absorption of nutrients once the feeding tube is placed distally. Fistulas located in the duodenum, distal ileum, or colon have higher success rates with enteral nutrition. Parental nutrition may be required for feeding intolerance or with high output fistulas.

17. C: A patient with gastroparesis who is unsuccessful in managing symptoms with an oral diet will need an alternate plan for medical nutrition therapy. There is still continued discussion regarding the optimal method for feeding a patient with gastroparesis. General consensus is for a trial of nasojejunal feeding while the patient is strictly NPO in order to determine if any intolerance is due to oral intake or tube feedings. A polymeric formula can be initiated because the stomach is bypassed. Fiber-containing formulas may not be tolerated as well due to abdominal discomfort and dysmotility. If tolerance is established, permanent jejunal access can be attained. Sometimes vented tubes are used in order to allow gastric venting for nausea and/or vomiting while feeding into the jejunum. Patients who are malnourished should be monitored closely for refeeding syndrome as enteral nutrition advances. Parenteral nutrition is typically the last choice for gastroparesis unless there is a complication involving both the stomach and the small bowel, such as a pseudo-obstruction.

18. B: An obstructed feeding tube can occur for many reasons, including medications administered through the tube, medications that are acidic or alkaline, inadequate flushing of the tube, or interaction of the formula with acid in the stomach. It is extremely important to try to maintain the patency of a feeding tube before clogging occurs. Tubes should be flushed with water every 4 hours, and whenever a tube is held or a medication is administered. Use of warm water irrigation is helpful in clearing an obstruction. The use of excessive pressure is not recommended because this may damage or rupture the tube. The use of cranberry juice or cola products have not been shown to have any advantage over water flushes. The next step should be flushing the tube with a mixture of pancreatic enzymes and water or sodium bicarbonate. Using a stiff wire is not recommended due to the risk of perforation.

19. A: Ciprofloxacin (Cipro) is a fluoroquinolone antibiotic. The bioavailability in this class of antibiotics is affected by the enteral formulation and route of formulation. Patients who receive Cipro via a J tube may have up to 82% loss of bioavailability of the drug. This may be due in part to the site of absorption and the binding of divalent cations such as calcium, magnesium, and iron to the enteral formula. For a patient receiving Cipro through the feeding tube, the tablet should be crushed and mixed into up to 60 mL of sterile water. The tube feeding is held for a minimum of 1 hour before and 2 hours after the medication is administered to improve bioavailability. Cipro suspension should not be administered through a feeding tube because clogging of the tube is likely. The rate of the tube feeding will need to be readjusted to account for the holding of the tube-feeding.

20. B: A chyle leak can be a difficult condition to manage. Chyle leaks can be caused by many reasons, including congenital lymphangiectasia, lymphoma, postoperative complications for radical neck dissections, pancreatic resections or other surgeries, or trauma to the chest or abdomen. Pleural fluid containing greater than 100 mg/dL of triglycerides would be indicative of a chyle leak. If a chest tube is placed and output is greater than 500 mL/day in adults, then TPN should be initiated. Lipids can be provided because the lymphatic system is not required and will not affect chyle flow. If the output is less than 500 mL per day, a low-fat elemental formula should be selected with medium-chain triglycerides (MCT) as the added fat source. MCTs are absorbed through the portal system and do not require the lymphatic system like long-chain fatty acids do. Indicators of tolerance to enteral nutrition would be a decrease in chest tube output. Surgery may be required if conservative treatment is required longer than 2 weeks.

21. A: Long-term total parenteral nutrition (TPN) may be indicated for a few conditions such massive small bowel resection, intensive chemotherapy, and other reasons. For patients requiring long-term TPN, a change to a cyclic schedule is often recommended in order to give the patient time away from the infusion pump. Cyclic TPN may also reduce the risk of liver complications associated with long-term TPN. The best candidates for this type of schedule would be stable patients who are not ventilated, those requiring intensive rehabilitative services such as physical or occupational therapy, or patients who will be receiving home TPN. The patients who are less likely to be candidates include those under the age of 3 (especially neonates with low glycogen reserves), patients with sensitive fluid issues such as congestive heart failure (CHF), and patients with uncontrolled blood sugar requiring insulin drips or long-acting insulin. A history of hypoglycemia would not preclude opportunity for cyclic TPN as long as blood glucose is monitored closely and the rate is tapered before discontinuation.

22. D: Patients with head and neck cancer will frequently have some type of feeding tube placed either before or during surgery depending upon the treatment plan. In this case, because chemotherapy and radiation are planned prior to surgery, a portacath needed to be placed for chemotherapy administration and at the same time, a PEJ was placed. A feeding tube in the jejunum is a good choice because it will help to reduce the risk of aspiration and the tube is placed below the potential surgical site. This patient's GI function appears to be within normal limits, so an elemental formula is not required. Most patients can tolerate isotonic fiber-containing formula delivered into the jejunum at full strength without difficulty. Generally, a low rate can be initiated and if the patient is tolerating the formula without problem, the rate can be increased every few hours up to goal. In a PEJ tube, the recommendations for increases vary between 6 to 12 hours. Bolus feedings are contraindicated with jejunal feeding tubes.

23. C: The TPN solution of 390 grams of dextrose and 70 grams protein in 1550 mL with 250 mL of lipids provides this patient with approximately 2106 kcal. She is receiving 1.2 grams/kg protein, 0.8 grams/kg lipid, and 36 kcal/kg. The glucose infusion rate is 4.6 mg/kg/minute. The solution is approximately 63% dextrose, 13% protein, and 24% lipid. The recommendations for this patient would be approximately 30 kcal/kg, 1.2-1.5 grams/ kg protein, 20-40% of total calories from lipids, and 40-60% of total calories from dextrose. Based on this information, the patient is likely being both overfed and receiving excessive dextrose as evidenced by hyperglycemia. The best action would be to reduce total calories and dextrose. A change to a solution of 250 cc 20% lipids with 290 grams dextrose and 70 grams protein in 1550 cc would provide 1766 kcal (30 kcal/kg) and reduce the glucose infusion rate to 3.4 mg/kg/minute. The solution would be 56% dextrose, 16% protein, 28% lipid.

24. B: Given that the patient had moderate malnutrition in the pre-transplant period, it is best not to discontinue enteral nutrition too quickly. Calorie needs post-transplant are not significantly elevated in the post-transplant period; however, sufficient calories are required for repletion and for the patient to be able to regain strength to perform activities of daily living and physical therapy. Protein needs are elevated in the immediate post-transplant period at approximately 1.5-2.0 grams/kg due to corticosteroids and healing. Once the patient is meeting at least 50% of her nutritional needs orally, the tube feeding schedule can be changed to nocturnal feedings to allow her oral intake to improve. Close monitoring of laboratory data and of calorie and protein intake and weight should also continue.

25. D: The patient's own wishes would take precedence in the determination for artificial nutrition and hydration (ANH); however, a patient with advanced dementia would not be able to make this decision in their current state. An advance directive such as a living will, written at a time when the patient was of sound mind, would take precedence over the surrogate decision maker, health care proxy, power of attorney, or close family member. A living will is a legal document that provides specific written instructions for making end-of-life decisions if the person is unable to do so. Durable power of attorney or health care proxy is also an advance directive that designates a specific person to make decisions in the event the patient is unable to. A surrogate decision maker is appointed by the court to act as a surrogate in making decisions if there is no other advance directive available.

26. C: Hypernatremia is an elevation in serum sodium level above 145 mEq/L. Many patients develop hypernatremia as a result of other conditions affecting fluid status. Unresolved hypernatremia can be extremely dangerous and can result in death. Patients at the highest risk for developing this disorder include elderly patients, infants, patients with a change in mental status, and those on mechanical ventilation. The majority of patients with hypernatremia will have a deficit of free water within the body. There are many different equations that can be used for evaluating the free water deficit. The factor used to estimate the total body water also varies. The equation to follow assumes a factor of 60% total body water. The equation also estimates 140 mEq/L as the normal serum sodium level. Water deficit (L) = 0.6 x body weight in kg [(actual serum sodium in mEq/L / 140 mEq/L) - 1]. Using the body weight of 80 kg and serum sodium of 156 mEq/L, the estimated water deficit is 5.28 liters.

27. A: Diarrhea is a common occurrence for patients receiving enteral nutrition. A standard definition of diarrhea has not been adopted universally. A general definition is more than 500 mL of stool every 8 hours or more than 3 stools in a 24-hour period for 3 days in a row. Measurement of stool volume can be a difficult task. One method for incontinent hospitalized patients is to use a pad on the bed, which can be weighed before and after bowel movements. The assumption is 1 gram of weight is equivalent to 1 mL of stool. Diarrhea can be caused by many different factors. These include antibiotics, magnesium-containing medications, laxatives, and stool softeners. Medications in the elixir form may also be a cause due to sorbitol as an additive which causes an osmotic diarrhea. *C. difficile* is a very common occurrence in hospitalized patients and should be verified. One treatment for diarrhea can be the inclusion of soluble fiber either in the tube feeding or as a medication such as Metamucil.

28. C: Hypertriglyceridemia is a risk for patients who are receiving central TPN as well as IV propofol (Diprivan) due to the potential for overfeeding dextrose and IV lipids. Propofol is a lipid-based sedative used in the ICU for the sedation of intubated patients. This medication is mixed in a 10% lipid emulsion and provides 1.1 kcal/cc and can contribute a significant amount of fat in certain cases. Hypertriglyceridemia is defined as a serum triglyceride level above 400 mg/dL. Untreated hypertriglyceridemia can lead to an altered immune response and pancreatitis if the levels rise above 1000 mg/dL. IV lipids should be limited to less than 30% of total calories or 1 g/kg or less per day. The IV lipid infusion rate should not be more than 0.11 grams/kg/hour. The glucose infusion rate should be less than 4-5 mg/kg/minute. If serum triglyceride levels are elevated, lipid intake and dextrose infusion from all sources should be closely evaluated.

29. B: The main metabolic responses to the refeeding syndrome are alterations in glucose metabolism, alterations in fluid and sodium balance, hypophosphatemia, hypokalemia, hypomagnesemia, and a deficiency in thiamine. A surge in insulin secretion in response to carbohydrate provision to a malnourished patient can cause an intracellular shift in phosphorus, potassium, and magnesium. These deficiencies can result in dangerous respiratory, cardiac, and neurological consequences. Phosphorus, potassium, and magnesium are all involved in multiple metabolic pathways including those requiring ATP as an intermediate. The sodium and fluid retention occur secondary to excessive insulin secretion coupled with insulin resistance (not SIADH). This leads to the simultaneous states of hyperglycemia and hyperinsulinemia, which result in sodium and fluid retention due to the effect of insulin on the renal tubules causing an antidiuretic effect. The sodium and fluid retention then leads to an expansion in extracellular volume, which in turn can cause pulmonary edema and cardiac failure. Thiamine deficiency can be exacerbated by additional demands for thiamine in response to an increase in glucose load. It is essential to monitor glucose and electrolyte levels closely for at least the first 3 days after initiation of nutrition therapy.

30. D: Metabolic alkalosis is a condition characterized by excessive hydrogen loss or excessive amounts of an alkaline substance such as bicarbonate (HCO_3^-). This can occur as a result of severe vomiting or hydrogen loss from the GI tract through nasogastric suction. Metabolic alkalosis is reflected by an increase in arterial pH and an increase in plasma HCO_3^-. The PCO_2 (or the amount of carbon dioxide in the blood) will increase as a result of the resultant hypoventilation. Gastric juices contain hydrogen chloride. Normally, hydrogen chloride from gastric juices will stimulate bicarbonate secretion when the acid reaches the duodenum. This process does not occur if the hydrogen chloride is lost from the GI tract. Metabolic alkalosis can also occur as a result of diuretic therapy. It can occur after a patient is treated aggressively for metabolic acidosis with either too much bicarbonate or the addition of too much acetate in the PN solution. Normally the kidneys can correct metabolic alkalosis by excreting the HCO_3^- in the urine.

31. B: Respiratory acidosis occurs when there is a decrease in alveolar ventilation. This is most often a result of obstructive lung disease such as chronic bronchitis or emphysema. It can also be a result of anesthesia or over-sedation, or as a result of a head injury or neuromuscular disorder such as myasthenia gravis. Laboratory values reflect an increase in PCO_2. This is known as hypercapnia or excessive carbon dioxide in the blood. Treatment is typically some type of bronchodilator medication, oxygen or positive pressure ventilation such as BiPAP. Patients who are obese should try to lose weight as this will aid in improved ventilation.

32. D: PN-associated liver disease (PNALD) can be a frequent occurrence in patients on long-term TPN. PNALD may manifest as cholestasis, steatosis, or gallbladder complications such as stones or sludge. PN-associated cholestasis occurs most often in children and is most often diagnosed with an elevation in alkaline phosphatase, GGT, and direct bilirubin levels. Cholestasis is a very serious condition because it may lead to liver failure requiring transplantation. Steatosis is may be evident with an increase in serum aminotransferase levels. Gallbladder complications may lead to cholecystitis. Clinical studies have shown that overfeeding of total calories, dextrose, and lipids may lead to liver complications. Excessive amino acid administration in infants may be an issue but it is less likely to lead to complications in adults. There are other non-nutritional causes that may be a factor in PNALD, such as hepatotoxic medications or biliary obstruction. Balancing the TPN solution, reducing lipid intake to less than 1 gram/kg, and reducing dextrose concentration are all steps to take initially.

33. C: The risk for pulmonary aspiration is highest in patients who are unconscious, in a supine position, intubated, and have delayed gastric emptying. Patients who are actively vomiting and who have a history of both aspiration and neuromuscular issues are also at risk. The best initial step to reduce the risk for pulmonary aspiration is to elevate the head of the bed to 45 degrees. Adding food coloring to the formula is no longer recommended and is associated with bacterial contamination, allergic reactions, and other complications. Monitoring gastric residuals is typically standard practice; however, agreement has not been reached on the level of residuals that indicates danger. A trend in gastric residuals may be helpful for monitoring purposes. There is no indication that a change in the type of formula would prevent aspiration. A post-pylorus feeding tube placed in the distal duodenum or proximal jejunum may be indicated.

34. A: Iron deficiency in a patient receiving long-term TPN may develop after the body stores of iron are depleted. This may occur around 6 months without an iron source. Oral supplementation may be provided with a functioning GI tract. Iron dextran cannot be added to total nutrient admixtures (also known as 3-in-1 solutions) because the iron dextran causes the lipid emulsion to become unstable and separate, making the admixture unsafe for administration. Manufacturers of the other 2 types of parenteral iron supplements (iron sucrose and sodium ferric gluconate) do not recommend this practice either because of the uncertainty surrounding safety. Iron dextran can be added to TPN solutions that do not contain lipids. Iron dextran can also be given intravenously. Anytime iron dextran is selected as the iron supplement, a test dose must be given due to the potential for a dangerous anaphylactic reaction. Parenteral iron should never be given to anyone with an infection because it may interfere with immune function and may promote bacterial growth.

35. B: Catheter-related occlusion is one of the most common complications of parenteral access devices. There are many reasons for occlusions, including mechanical obstruction, lipid emulsions, and precipitates of calcium or phosphate from the solution, but the main reason is due to a blood clot. If a blood clot is present but untreated, it can lead to complete occlusion or blockage of the vein or artery. A line is considered occluded when it is difficult to infuse into the line or to aspirate blood from the line. This can happen if the line is not sufficiently flushed after blood is withdrawn. Initial symptoms of catheter-related thrombosis are frequent pump alarms or difficulty or inability to infuse through or aspirate from the line. As the symptoms advance, swelling around the eyes, face, and neck may occur. The arm may also swell and become discolored. Rapid heart rate and shortness of breath may also be clinically present. A physical examination and an ultrasound or venogram is needed to diagnose.

36. C: Symptoms of tube displacement include nausea, vomiting, and abdominal pain. The presence of a choking feeling or difficulty breathing is also a symptom and may be a result of an NG tube that has migrated from the stomach into the throat. If a tube dislodgment is suspected, the tube feeding should be stopped immediately. If the tube has been placed nasally, the tube should be pulled out. If the tube has been placed percutaneously, the tube should not be removed unless instructed to do so by the physician. Tube displacement can occur if the tube is not secured appropriately or if nausea and vomiting are persistent. It may also occur if the balloon that is holding the tube in place has been deflated. The length of the tube should be monitored before each feeding. A mark on the tube 1 inch from the entrance point will help to determine if the tube has migrated.

37. D: The main goal in the initiation of nutrition support in a patient at risk for the refeeding syndrome is to start slowly. The provision of excessive caloric intake could potentially cause death in a severely malnourished patient. There are various recommendations in the literature for determining the appropriate starting point for calories. These recommendations vary from 1000 kcals per day to 15-120 kcal/kg to 20% above BEE to 50% of calculated energy requirements using the Harris Benedict equation plus a factor of 1.3-1.5. The patient's actual weight should be used for calculations. Fluid and sodium intake should also be started slowly. The most important aspect of initiation is to monitor electrolyte levels, especially potassium, phosphorus, and magnesium, and aggressively replenish to prevent serious metabolic consequences. Glucose should also be monitored closely and controlled because the state of catabolism will not improve until glucose levels are under control. Uncontrolled glucose levels may also delay the refeeding response, causing additional complications.

38. A: Patients receiving long-term TPN are at high risk for the development of metabolic bone disease. This is diagnosed using DEXA (dual energy x-ray absorptiometry). There are many factors involved in the development of PN-associated metabolic bone disease. Non-nutritional factors include immobilization or prolonged bed rest, cigarette smoking, and alcohol abuse. Nutritional factors include inadequate negative calcium balance. Calcium balance is complicated. Increases in urinary calcium loss can be caused by higher calcium doses, high protein intake (especially greater than 2 grams/kg), and insufficient phosphorus intake. Calcium should be provided at 10-15 mEq per day and phosphorus at 20-40 mmol per day. Prevention of metabolic acidosis is also important with the addition of acetate to the solution. Cycling the PN solution also reduces urinary calcium losses. Magnesium deficiency can also be a factor in metabolic bone disease and 8-20 mEq per day should be provided as a dose. Vitamin D deficiency should be corrected.

39. C: Once a patient is home from the hospital, their medical condition tends to be more stable. Initially, labs need to be checked once or twice in the first week. If the lab data is within normal limits, then monitoring can transition to weekly, then every 2 weeks, then monthly as a pattern of stability is established. Some long-term TPN patients can be monitored once or twice per year. The lab data that should be included is the comprehensive metabolic panel including electrolytes, BUN, creatinine, liver function tests, calcium, phosphorus, magnesium, albumin, and complete blood count with differential. A baseline triglyceride and PT/PTT/INR should be obtained; then these can be checked monthly or as needed. Iron studies should be obtained twice per year. A yearly assessment of vitamin and mineral status, including vitamins A, D, and E, and selenium, zinc, manganese, and copper is prudent. Bone density should also be measured annually.

40. B: Vitamin D is a fat-soluble vitamin. It can be obtained from certain foods such as dairy products, supplements, or ultraviolet rays. Vitamin D must go through 2 hydroxylations before it reaches the active form of vitamin D. The first hydroxylation happens in the liver, where vitamin D is converted to 25-hydroxyvitamin D ([25-(OH)D]) or calcidiol. The next step occurs in the kidney, where calcidiol is converted to the active form 1,25-dihydroxyvitamin D [1,25-$(OH)_2D$]. This is known as calcitriol. Individuals with impaired kidney function may have trouble converting vitamin D to the active form when the glomerular filtration rate declines below 20 mL/minute and when PTH levels are elevated above 300 pg/mL. Serum 25-(OH)D levels are the best indicator of vitamin D. 1,25-$(OH)_2D$ is not as good of an indicator because it has a very short half-life of 15 hours and its levels are very closely regulated by PTH, calcium, and phosphate levels. 1,25-$(OH)_2D$ levels do not usually fall until a severe vitamin D deficiency has developed.

41. A: Omeprazole is a proton pump inhibitor used in the treatment of gastroesophageal reflux disease (GERD). It is an enteric-coated, delayed-release medication. The enteric coating protects the medication until it reaches the alkaline pH of the duodenum, where the capsule is fully dissolved and absorbed. If the medication must be given through an NG tube, G tube, or PEG, it must be altered. This medication cannot be crushed because it will clog the feeding tube and it will not be able to be absorbed in the small intestine. The granules must stay intact. The granules should be mixed with an acidic fruit juice such as apple, orange, or cranberry, then flushed with additional juice. The feeding should be held for an hour to ensure absorption.

42. D: The main route of excretion for manganese and copper is through the biliary system. Elevated manganese levels are more likely in patients who have elevated bilirubin levels. Elevated manganese levels can also be seen in patients on long-term TPN without toxicity symptoms. Levels should be monitored at baseline, then every 3 months unless the bilirubin is elevated. In this case, levels should be checked monthly. Manganese should be removed from the TPN solution if manganese levels are elevated. Toxicity symptoms may include neurologic events such as headache, tremors, and alterations in gait. For patients with cholestasis, copper should be reduced or removed from the TPN solution. Serum levels should be checked monthly and signs of deficiency, such as hypochromic microcytic anemia, neutropenia, and skeletal abnormalities should be watched for. Trace elements are typically added in a single product that includes chromium, copper, manganese, zinc, and selenium. Single additives of trace elements are available to add separately when required.

43. B: Protocols for PPN should be written for the safety of patients receiving this type of nutrition support therapy. Generally, patients who are good candidates for PPN include those with good peripheral veins for placement of the peripheral catheter who will be able to tolerate a large amount of fluid. Therapy for PPN is limited to 2 weeks or less due to access issues and tolerance to PPN solutions. The osmolarity of PPN solutions should be less than 900 mOsm/L and are usually comprised of dextrose concentration of 5-10% and final amino acid concentration of 3%. Solutions with an osmolarity greater than 900 mOsm/L should be infused through a central vein. A midline catheter is a longer peripheral line that is placed in a larger vein but is still considered peripheral. Peripheral lines or cannulas should be rotated every 72 hours to reduce the risk for phlebitis. Research has shown that phlebitis is more likely on the fourth day of PPN.

44. A: Prevention of catheter-related infection is extremely important due to the risk of sepsis. A written policy and procedure should be in place utilizing the current EBM. The proper care of the catheter and insertion site is pivotal. Appropriate antiseptic agents include chlorhexidine, tincture of iodine, and 70% alcohol. Antibiotic creams or ointments such as Neosporin or Bacitracin are contraindicated due to the risk of fungal infections. Catheter sites should be checked every day to observe for redness, tenderness, or other signs of infection. Water should not be used around the insertion site to decrease the risk of microorganisms entering the site. A schedule for dressing changes should be established based on the type of dressing used. For example, a transparent dressing on a tunneled central venous catheter should be changed once per week until healing of the insertion site is complete, unless there are indications that the dressing should be changed sooner.

45. D: The use of the femoral artery is the least preferred site for CVC insertion due to the risk for infection and thrombosis. The subclavian is the preferred site. The internal jugular is another site frequently used for CVC. The basilic, cephalic, and brachial sites are the vessels used for placement of a PICC (peripherally inserted central venous catheter). The use of a tunneled catheter, such as a Broviac, helps to decrease the risk of infection because there is a separation between the exit and the venipuncture site. These are used frequently for long-term TPN and CVC access required at home. An implanted catheter is a port placed within a subcutaneous pocket and is less visible than other types of CVC. This type of CVC is used frequently for chemotherapy administration.

46. C: The Patient Self-Determination Act is a federal law passed in 1990. The law was enacted as a way to help patients understand their health care rights and to aid in decision-making. The law requires that it is the responsibility of the healthcare institution to advise patients of their rights and to determine if there is an advance directive already established. If there is such a document, it must be documented in the patient's medical record that the advance directive exists. The law does not require a hard copy of the advanced directive to be available and it does not require that all patients have an advance directive. A health care advance directive is a general term used to define any written statements regarding future health care decisions. An advance directive would include a living will and a health care power of attorney. Instructions to be included in the document would be the type of care desired in various health care situations, such as dementia or persistent vegetative state.

47. A: The provision of artificial nutrition and hydration (ANH) is a complicated area and ASPEN has written a position paper on this topic. There are cases in which ANH may not be advisable, including severe advanced dementia, persistent vegetative state, and some terminal illnesses. ANH has been shown to add risks or complications to certain patients with an increase in nausea, vomiting, or aspiration pneumonia. In these cases, risks may outweigh the benefits of ANH. Although it is difficult to make any decision to withhold or forgo ANH, it is especially difficult in the pediatric population. This decision is usually a joint decision between the parents and medical team when continuing ANH may be a burden to the child. Cultural aspects should be considered for all patients including religious and ethnic factors. ASPEN guidelines also state that health care professionals should not be forced to provide ANH if the health care provider believes the therapy is contraindicated. If there is any conflict surrounding nutrition, ANH should be continued until the conflict is resolved.

48. B: Evidence-based practice utilizes up-to-date research to apply to current practice. It is imperative that the research used was a well-designed study. The gold standard for research is the randomized controlled trial (RCT). This type of research has the least amount of bias within the study design and can produce honest, straightforward results. If RCT is not available, the next type of research to use would be a non-randomized, well-designed controlled study. This would be followed by cohort or case-controlled analytic studies. The type of research that is least appropriate for use in EBP is meta-analysis, review articles, or consensus statements. It is difficult to stay abreast of current research but tools are available to help with this. Two examples of tools are clinical evidence and *The Physician's Information and Education Resource* from the American College of Physician's. Other tools include *UpToDate* and *Harrison's Principles of Internal Medicine.*

49. C: There are only a few clinical trials studying the use of branched-chain amino acids in the treatment of encephalopathy. These studies have a very small number of patients and have not been able to prove the efficacy of this treatment for encephalopathy. The best EBP is to save formulas containing branched-chain amino acids for those patients who are not responding to aggressive medical management after all other efforts have been tried. These formulas are very expensive and their use has not been supported by research. The patient in question may be encephalopathic due to dehydration or nonadherent with lactulose therapy. Other causes of encephalopathy include GI bleeding, constipation or diarrhea, and use of narcotic or benzodiazepine medications.

50. D: The Joint Commission (TJC), formerly known as the Joint Commission on Accreditation of Healthcare Organizations, defines a sentinel event as "an unexpected occurrence involving death or serious injury or psychological injury or the risk thereof." A serious injury may result in the loss of an extremity or loss of function in some way. These occurrences are referred to as sentinel because immediate and emergent action is required for investigation. A rapid response is also required. An insulin overdose would be considered a sentinel event. Each health care institution must have its own policies and procedures surrounding a sentinel event, including root cause analysis and an action plan. Some sentinel events are referred to as reviewable or non-reviewable and each has specific steps involved in the response to the event. Health care institutions are encouraged but not mandated to report sentinel events to TJC. However, if TJC investigates an incident it hears about, the minimum expectation is that appropriate steps were taken in resolution of the event.

How to Overcome Test Anxiety

Just the thought of taking a test is enough to make most people a little nervous. A test is an important event that can have a long-term impact on your future, so it's important to take it seriously and it's natural to feel anxious about performing well. But just because anxiety is normal, that doesn't mean that it's helpful in test taking, or that you should simply accept it as part of your life. Anxiety can have a variety of effects. These effects can be mild, like making you feel slightly nervous, or severe, like blocking your ability to focus or remember even a simple detail.

If you experience test anxiety—whether severe or mild—it's important to know how to beat it. To discover this, first you need to understand what causes test anxiety.

Causes of Test Anxiety

While we often think of anxiety as an uncontrollable emotional state, it can actually be caused by simple, practical things. One of the most common causes of test anxiety is that a person does not feel adequately prepared for their test. This feeling can be the result of many different issues such as poor study habits or lack of organization, but the most common culprit is time management. Starting to study too late, failing to organize your study time to cover all of the material, or being distracted while you study will mean that you're not well prepared for the test. This may lead to cramming the night before, which will cause you to be physically and mentally exhausted for the test. Poor time management also contributes to feelings of stress, fear, and hopelessness as you realize you are not well prepared but don't know what to do about it.

Other times, test anxiety is not related to your preparation for the test but comes from unresolved fear. This may be a past failure on a test, or poor performance on tests in general. It may come from comparing yourself to others who seem to be performing better or from the stress of living up to expectations. Anxiety may be driven by fears of the future—how failure on this test would affect your educational and career goals. These fears are often completely irrational, but they can still negatively impact your test performance.

Elements of Test Anxiety

As mentioned earlier, test anxiety is considered to be an emotional state, but it has physical and mental components as well. Sometimes you may not even realize that you are suffering from test anxiety until you notice the physical symptoms. These can include trembling hands, rapid heartbeat, sweating, nausea, and tense muscles. Extreme anxiety may lead to fainting or vomiting. Obviously, any of these symptoms can have a negative impact on testing. It is important to recognize them as soon as they begin to occur so that you can address the problem before it damages your performance.

The mental components of test anxiety include trouble focusing and inability to remember learned information. During a test, your mind is on high alert, which can help you recall information and stay focused for an extended period of time. However, anxiety interferes with your mind's natural processes, causing you to blank out, even on the questions you know well. The strain of testing during anxiety makes it difficult to stay focused, especially on a test that may take several hours. Extreme anxiety can take a huge mental toll, making it difficult not only to recall test information but even to understand the test questions or pull your thoughts together.

Effects of Test Anxiety

Test anxiety is like a disease—if left untreated, it will get progressively worse. Anxiety leads to poor performance, and this reinforces the feelings of fear and failure, which in turn lead to poor performances on subsequent tests. It can grow from a mild nervousness to a crippling condition. If allowed to progress, test anxiety can have a big impact on your schooling, and consequently on your future.

Test anxiety can spread to other parts of your life. Anxiety on tests can become anxiety in any stressful situation, and blanking on a test can turn into panicking in a job situation. But fortunately, you don't have to let anxiety rule your testing and determine your grades. There are a number of relatively simple steps you can take to move past anxiety and function normally on a test and in the rest of life.

Physical Steps for Beating Test Anxiety

While test anxiety is a serious problem, the good news is that it can be overcome. It doesn't have to control your ability to think and remember information. While it may take time, you can begin taking steps today to beat anxiety.

Just as your first hint that you may be struggling with anxiety comes from the physical symptoms, the first step to treating it is also physical. Rest is crucial for having a clear, strong mind. If you are tired, it is much easier to give in to anxiety. But if you establish good sleep habits, your body and mind will be ready to perform optimally, without the strain of exhaustion. Additionally, sleeping well helps you to retain information better, so you're more likely to recall the answers when you see the test questions.

Getting good sleep means more than going to bed on time. It's important to allow your brain time to relax. Take study breaks from time to time so it doesn't get overworked, and don't study right before bed. Take time to rest your mind before trying to rest your body, or you may find it difficult to fall asleep.

Along with sleep, other aspects of physical health are important in preparing for a test. Good nutrition is vital for good brain function. Sugary foods and drinks may give a burst of energy but this burst is followed by a crash, both physically and emotionally. Instead, fuel your body with protein and vitamin-rich foods.

Also, drink plenty of water. Dehydration can lead to headaches and exhaustion, especially if your brain is already under stress from the rigors of the test. Particularly if your test is a long one, drink water during the breaks. And if possible, take an energy-boosting snack to eat between sections.

Along with sleep and diet, a third important part of physical health is exercise. Maintaining a steady workout schedule is helpful, but even taking 5-minute study breaks to walk can help get your blood pumping faster and clear your head. Exercise also releases endorphins, which contribute to a positive feeling and can help combat test anxiety.

When you nurture your physical health, you are also contributing to your mental health. If your body is healthy, your mind is much more likely to be healthy as well. So take time to rest, nourish your body with healthy food and water, and get moving as much as possible. Taking these physical steps will make you stronger and more able to take the mental steps necessary to overcome test anxiety.

Mental Steps for Beating Test Anxiety

Working on the mental side of test anxiety can be more challenging, but as with the physical side, there are clear steps you can take to overcome it. As mentioned earlier, test anxiety often stems from lack of preparation, so the obvious solution is to prepare for the test. Effective studying may be the most important weapon you have for beating test anxiety, but you can and should employ several other mental tools to combat fear.

First, boost your confidence by reminding yourself of past success—tests or projects that you aced. If you're putting as much effort into preparing for this test as you did for those, there's no reason you should expect to fail here. Work hard to prepare; then trust your preparation.

Second, surround yourself with encouraging people. It can be helpful to find a study group, but be sure that the people you're around will encourage a positive attitude. If you spend time with others who are anxious or cynical, this will only contribute to your own anxiety. Look for others who are motivated to study hard from a desire to succeed, not from a fear of failure.

Third, reward yourself. A test is physically and mentally tiring, even without anxiety, and it can be helpful to have something to look forward to. Plan an activity following the test, regardless of the outcome, such as going to a movie or getting ice cream.

When you are taking the test, if you find yourself beginning to feel anxious, remind yourself that you know the material. Visualize successfully completing the test. Then take a few deep, relaxing breaths and return to it. Work through the questions carefully but with confidence, knowing that you are capable of succeeding.

Developing a healthy mental approach to test taking will also aid in other areas of life. Test anxiety affects more than just the actual test—it can be damaging to your mental health and even contribute to depression. It's important to beat test anxiety before it becomes a problem for more than testing.

Study Strategy

Being prepared for the test is necessary to combat anxiety, but what does being prepared look like? You may study for hours on end and still not feel prepared. What you need is a strategy for test prep. The next few pages outline our recommended steps to help you plan out and conquer the challenge of preparation.

Step 1: Scope Out the Test

Learn everything you can about the format (multiple choice, essay, etc.) and what will be on the test. Gather any study materials, course outlines, or sample exams that may be available. Not only will this help you to prepare, but knowing what to expect can help to alleviate test anxiety.

Step 2: Map Out the Material

Look through the textbook or study guide and make note of how many chapters or sections it has. Then divide these over the time you have. For example, if a book has 15 chapters and you have five days to study, you need to cover three chapters each day. Even better, if you have the time, leave an extra day at the end for overall review after you have gone through the material in depth.

If time is limited, you may need to prioritize the material. Look through it and make note of which sections you think you already have a good grasp on, and which need review. While you are studying, skim quickly through the familiar sections and take more time on the challenging parts. Write out your plan so you don't get lost as you go. Having a written plan also helps you feel more in control of the study, so anxiety is less likely to arise from feeling overwhelmed at the amount to cover.

Step 3: Gather Your Tools

Decide what study method works best for you. Do you prefer to highlight in the book as you study and then go back over the highlighted portions? Or do you type out notes of the important information? Or is it helpful to make flashcards that you can carry with you? Assemble the pens, index cards, highlighters, post-it notes, and any other materials you may need so you won't be distracted by getting up to find things while you study.

If you're having a hard time retaining the information or organizing your notes, experiment with different methods. For example, try color-coding by subject with colored pens, highlighters, or post-it notes. If you learn better by hearing, try recording yourself reading your notes so you can listen while in the car, working out, or simply sitting at your desk. Ask a friend to quiz you from your flashcards, or try teaching someone the material to solidify it in your mind.

Step 4: Create Your Environment

It's important to avoid distractions while you study. This includes both the obvious distractions like visitors and the subtle distractions like an uncomfortable chair (or a too-comfortable couch that makes you want to fall asleep). Set up the best study environment possible: good lighting and a comfortable work area. If background music helps you focus, you may want to turn it on, but otherwise keep the room quiet. If you are using a computer to take notes, be sure you don't have any other windows open, especially applications like social media, games, or anything else that could distract you. Silence your phone and turn off notifications. Be sure to keep water close by so you stay hydrated while you study (but avoid unhealthy drinks and snacks).

Also, take into account the best time of day to study. Are you freshest first thing in the morning? Try to set aside some time then to work through the material. Is your mind clearer in the afternoon or evening? Schedule your study session then. Another method is to study at the same time of day that you will take the test, so that your brain gets used to working on the material at that time and will be ready to focus at test time.

Step 5: Study!

Once you have done all the study preparation, it's time to settle into the actual studying. Sit down, take a few moments to settle your mind so you can focus, and begin to follow your study plan. Don't give in to distractions or let yourself procrastinate. This is your time to prepare so you'll be ready to fearlessly approach the test. Make the most of the time and stay focused.

Of course, you don't want to burn out. If you study too long you may find that you're not retaining the information very well. Take regular study breaks. For example, taking five minutes out of every hour to walk briskly, breathing deeply and swinging your arms, can help your mind stay fresh.

As you get to the end of each chapter or section, it's a good idea to do a quick review. Remind yourself of what you learned and work on any difficult parts. When you feel that you've mastered the material, move on to the next part. At the end of your study session, briefly skim through your notes again.

But while review is helpful, cramming last minute is NOT. If at all possible, work ahead so that you won't need to fit all your study into the last day. Cramming overloads your brain with more information than it can process and retain, and your tired mind may struggle to recall even previously learned information when it is overwhelmed with last-minute study. Also, the urgent nature of cramming and the stress placed on your brain contribute to anxiety. You'll be more likely to go to the test feeling unprepared and having trouble thinking clearly.

So don't cram, and don't stay up late before the test, even just to review your notes at a leisurely pace. Your brain needs rest more than it needs to go over the information again. In fact, plan to finish your studies by noon or early afternoon the day before the test. Give your brain the rest of the day to relax or focus on other things, and get a good night's sleep. Then you will be fresh for the test and better able to recall what you've studied.

Step 6: Take a Practice Test

Many courses offer sample tests, either online or in the study materials. This is an excellent resource to check whether you have mastered the material, as well as to prepare for the test format and environment.

Check the test format ahead of time: the number of questions, the type (multiple choice, free response, etc.), and the time limit. Then create a plan for working through them. For example, if you have 30 minutes to take a 60-question test, your limit is 30 seconds per question. Spend less time on the questions you know well so that you can take more time on the difficult ones.

If you have time to take several practice tests, take the first one open book, with no time limit. Work through the questions at your own pace and make sure you fully understand them. Gradually work up to taking a test under test conditions: sit at a desk with all study materials put away and set a timer. Pace yourself to make sure you finish the test with time to spare and go back to check your answers if you have time.

After each test, check your answers. On the questions you missed, be sure you understand why you missed them. Did you misread the question (tests can use tricky wording)? Did you forget the information? Or was it something you hadn't learned? Go back and study any shaky areas that the practice tests reveal.

Taking these tests not only helps with your grade, but also aids in combating test anxiety. If you're already used to the test conditions, you're less likely to worry about it, and working through tests until you're scoring well gives you a confidence boost. Go through the practice tests until you feel comfortable, and then you can go into the test knowing that you're ready for it.

Test Tips

On test day, you should be confident, knowing that you've prepared well and are ready to answer the questions. But aside from preparation, there are several test day strategies you can employ to maximize your performance.

First, as stated before, get a good night's sleep the night before the test (and for several nights before that, if possible). Go into the test with a fresh, alert mind rather than staying up late to study.

Try not to change too much about your normal routine on the day of the test. It's important to eat a nutritious breakfast, but if you normally don't eat breakfast at all, consider eating just a protein bar. If you're a coffee drinker, go ahead and have your normal coffee. Just make sure you time it so that the caffeine doesn't wear off right in the middle of your test. Avoid sugary beverages, and drink enough water to stay hydrated but not so much that you need a restroom break 10 minutes into the test. If your test isn't first thing in the morning, consider going for a walk or doing a light workout before the test to get your blood flowing.

Allow yourself enough time to get ready, and leave for the test with plenty of time to spare so you won't have the anxiety of scrambling to arrive in time. Another reason to be early is to select a good seat. It's helpful to sit away from doors and windows, which can be distracting. Find a good seat, get out your supplies, and settle your mind before the test begins.

When the test begins, start by going over the instructions carefully, even if you already know what to expect. Make sure you avoid any careless mistakes by following the directions.

Then begin working through the questions, pacing yourself as you've practiced. If you're not sure on an answer, don't spend too much time on it, and don't let it shake your confidence. Either skip it and come back later, or eliminate as many wrong answers as possible and guess among the remaining ones. Don't dwell on these questions as you continue—put them out of your mind and focus on what lies ahead.

Be sure to read all of the answer choices, even if you're sure the first one is the right answer. Sometimes you'll find a better one if you keep reading. But don't second-guess yourself if you do immediately know the answer. Your gut instinct is usually right. Don't let test anxiety rob you of the information you know.

If you have time at the end of the test (and if the test format allows), go back and review your answers. Be cautious about changing any, since your first instinct tends to be correct, but make sure you didn't misread any of the questions or accidentally mark the wrong answer choice. Look over any you skipped and make an educated guess.

At the end, leave the test feeling confident. You've done your best, so don't waste time worrying about your performance or wishing you could change anything. Instead, celebrate the successful completion of this test. And finally, use this test to learn how to deal with anxiety even better next time.

Review Video: Test Anxiety
Visit mometrix.com/academy and enter code: 100340

Important Qualification

Not all anxiety is created equal. If your test anxiety is causing major issues in your life beyond the classroom or testing center, or if you are experiencing troubling physical symptoms related to your anxiety, it may be a sign of a serious physiological or psychological condition. If this sounds like your situation, we strongly encourage you to seek professional help.

Online Resources

Due to our efforts to try to keep this book to a manageable length, we've created a link that will give you access to all of your online resources:

mometrix.com/resources719/nutrition

It's Your Moment, Let's Celebrate It!

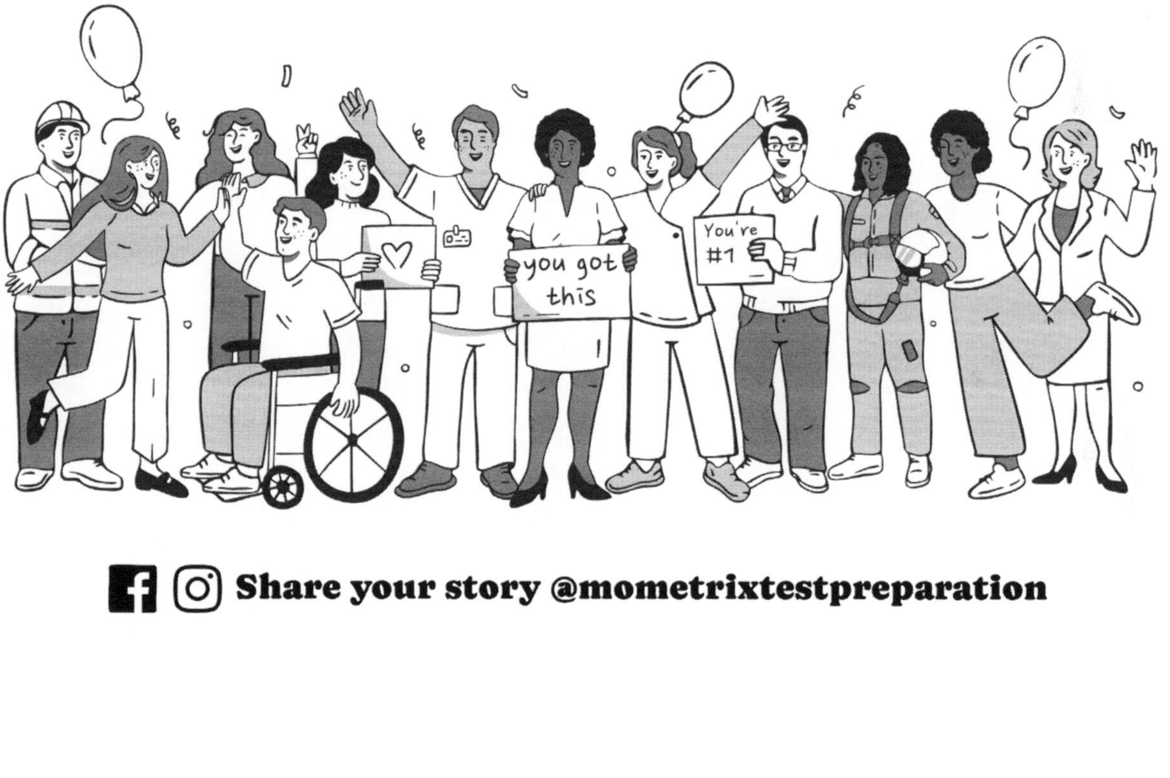

Share your story @mometrixtestpreparation